Sepsis and Organ Dysfunction
From Basics to Clinical Approach

A Tribute to Roger Bone

Springer

Milano
Berlin
Heidelberg
New York
Barcelona
Hong Kong
London
Paris
Singapore
Tokyo

A.E. Baue
G. Berlot
A. Gullo
J.-L. Vincent (Eds)

Sepsis and Organ Dysfunction

From Basics to Clinical Approach

ORGAN FAILURE ACADEMY

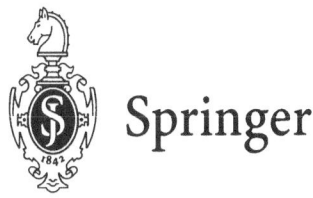

Springer

A.E. Baue M.D.
Department of Surgery, Saint Louis University, Health Sciences Center, St. Louis - USA

G. Berlot M.D.
Department of Anaesthesia, Intensive Care and Pain Therapy
University of Trieste, Cattinara Hospital, Trieste - Italy

A. Gullo M.D.
Department of Anaesthesia, Intensive Care and Pain Therapy
University of Trieste, Cattinara Hospital, Trieste - Italy

J.-L. Vincent M.D.
Department of Intensive Care, Erasme University Hospital
Free University of Brussels - Belgium

© Springer-Verlag Italia, Milano 1999

ISBN-13: 978-88-470-0052-0   e-ISBN-13: 978-88-470-2248-5
DOI: 10.1007/ 978-88-470-2248-5

Library of Congress Cataloging-in-Publication Data: Applied for

Cover design: Simona Colombo, Milan

SPIN : 10707117

A TRIBUTE TO ROGER BONE

Last year, intensive care medicine lost one of its leading proponents, but Roger Bone is not forgotten. Roger was a prominent and highly respected member of the international intensive care community who is remembered by many for his outstanding scientific contributions to intensive care medicine, particularly in the fields of sepsis and acute respiratory failure. Roger was an enthusiast, dedicated and committed to his chosen specialty and worked with endless enthusiasm and vision to promote and advance intensive care medicine both at home and abroad. As scientist, clinician, teacher, author and editor, Roger always found time to assist and support the work of his colleagues, willing to take time to listen and offer valuable comment and criticism. His opinions were always respected, even if we did not agree with all his scientific arguments, and his capability and commitment to intensive care medicine were never questioned.

Roger approached his final illness with remarkable fortitude and bravery, accepting the inevitable with courage and characteristically continuing his scientific and academic activities throughout, showing many that the process of dying is just the final part of living.

A charismatic and highly valued leader in intensive care medicine has been taken from us, but Roger Bone has left a great legacy as scientist, clinician, author, editor, lecturer, and friend – his memory will live on.

J.-L. Vincent

Table of Contents

Introduction
A.E. BAUE.. 13

BASIC PATHOPHYSIOLOGY MECHANICS

Inflammation: How Much Is Too Much and Can It Be Controlled?
V. RUMALLA, AND S.F. LOWRY.. 23

Injury, Inflammation, Sepsis - Is There a Natural, Organized and Sequential
Progression of Neuroendocrine, Metabolic and Cytokine Mediator Events Leading
to Organ System Failure?
A.E. BAUE.. 37

Genetic Predisposition to Sepsis and Organ Failure
B.A. ZEHNBAUER, B.D. FREEMAN, AND T.G. BUCHMAN.. 49

Regulation of the Lung Inflammatory Response
P.A. WARD, AND A.B. LENTSCH.. 55

CLINICAL INTERVENTIONS IN THE FIELD OF SEPSIS

WHAT IS WRONG AND WHAT IS RIGHT

Shall We Continue to Talk About (or Use) SIRS in the Twenty-first Century?
J.-L. VINCENT... 65

Prevention and Treatment of Sepsis - Present and Future Problems
A.E. BAUE.. 69

Sepsis and MODS - What Is Wrong and What Is Right
A. GULLO, AND G. BERLOT... 83

What Is Clinical Relevance? - Well Controlled Experiments in Normal Animals
as Compared to Clinical Studies in Diverse Sick Patients
A.E. BAUE.. 95

THE MARKERS OF SEPSIS

Apoptosis (Programmed Cell Death) and the Resolution of Acute Inflammation
A.H. ROUZATI, R. TANEJA, AND J.C. MARSHALL.. 107

"Untimely Apoptosis" Is the Password
T.G. BUCHMAN.. 117

Multiple Therapeutic Agents - Will Individual Therapies, Each of Which Improves Patients, When Given Together, Change Mortality?
A.E. BAUE 123

Endotoxaemia in Critical Illness: Rapid Detection and Clinical Relevance
J.C. MARSHALL, D.M. FOSTER, P.M. WALKER, AND A. ROMASCHIN 137

New and Old Markers in Sepsis
K. REINHART, AND W. KARZAI 147

From Cytokines through Immune Effector Cells to the Body
M.R. PINSKY 153

Intravenous Immunoglobulins: Are They Helpful?
G. PILZ 161

CLINICAL ASPECTS OF SPLANCHNIC ISCHAEMIA AND OXYGEN METABOLISM

Is Splanchnic Perfusion a Critical Problem in Sepsis?
M. POEZE, J.W.M. GREVE, AND G. RAMSAY 169

Metabolism and O_2 Consumption in Trauma and Sepsis
L. BRAZZI, P. PELOSI, AND L. GATTINONI 181

Intragastric pH (ipH) and $PaCO_2$ Monitoring in Sepsis
D. DE BACKER, J. CRETEUR, AND E. SILVA 187

Index 195

Authors Index

Baue A.E.
Dept. of Surgery, St. Louis University Health Sciences Centre, St. Louis, Missouri (U.S.A.)

Berlot G.
Dept. of Anaesthesiology and Intensive Care, Trieste University School of Medicine, Trieste (Italy)

Brazzi L.
Dept. of Anaesthesia and Intensive Care, Maggiore Hospital - IRCCS, Milan University School of Medicine, Milan (Italy)

Buchman T.G.
Dept. of Surgery, Anaesthesiology and Medicine, Washington University School of Medicine, St. Louis, Missouri (U.S.A.)

Creteur J.
Dept. of Intensive Care, Free University of Brussels, Erasme Hospital, Brussels (Belgium)

De Backer D.
Dept. of Intensive Care, Free University of Brussels, Erasme Hospital, Brussels (Belgium)

Freeman B.D.
Dept. of Surgery, Anaesthesiology and Medicine, Washington University School of Medicine, St. Louis, Missouri (U.S.A.)

Foster D.M.
General and Critical Care Surgery, Toronto Hospital, University of Toronto, Toronto, Ontario (Canada)

Gattinoni L.
Dept. of Anaesthesia and Intensive Care, Maggiore Hospital - IRCCS, Milan University School of Medicine, Milan (Italy)

Greve J.W.M.
Dept. of Surgery, Maastricht University Hospital, Maastricht (The Netherlands)

Gullo A.
Dept. of Anaesthesiology and Intensive Care, Trieste University School of Medicine, Trieste (Italy)

Karzai W.
Dept. of Anaesthesiology and Intensive Care, Friedrich Schiller University, Jena (Germany)

Lentsch A.B.
Dept. of Surgery, University of Louisville, Louisville, Kentucky (U.S.A.)

Lowry S.F.
Dept. of Surgery, University of Medicine and Dentistry of New Jersey, Robert Wood Johnson Medical School, New Brunswick, New Jersey (U.S.A.)

Marshall J.C.
General and Critical Care Surgery, Toronto Hospital, University of Toronto, Toronto, Ontario (Canada)

Pelosi P.
Dept. of Anaesthesia and Intensive Care, Maggiore Hospital - IRCCS, Milan University School of Medicine, Milan (Italy)

Pilz G.
Dept. of Medicine, Grosshadern Hospital, Ludwig-Maximilians University, München (Germany)

Pinsky M.R.
Division of Critical Care Medicine, Pittsburgh University, Pittsburgh, Pennsylvania (U.S.A.)

Poeze M.
Dept. of Surgery, Maastricht University Hospital, Maastricht (The Netherlands)

Ramsay G.
Dept. of Surgery, Maastricht University Hospital, Maastricht (The Netherlands)

Romaschin A.
General and Critical Care Surgery, Toronto Hospital, University of Toronto, Toronto, Ontario (Canada)

Rouzati A.H.
General and Critical Care Surgery, Toronto Hospital, University of Toronto, Toronto, Ontario (Canada)

Reinhart K.
Dept. of Anaesthesiology and Intensive Care, Friedrich Schiller University, Jena (Germany)

Rumalla V.
Dept. of Surgery, University of Medicine and Dentistry of New Jersey, Robert Wood Johnson Medical School, New Brunswick, New Jersey (U.S.A.)

Silva E.
Dept. of Intensive Care, Erasme University Hospital, Free University of Brussels, Brussels (Belgium)

Taneja R.
General and Critical Care Surgery, Toronto Hospital, University of Toronto, Toronto, Ontario (Canada)

Vincent J.-L.
Dept. of Intensive Care, Erasme University Hospital, Free University of Brussels, Brussels (Belgium)

Walker P.M.
General and Critical Care Surgery, Toronto Hospital, University of Toronto, Toronto, Ontario (Canada)

Ward P.A.
Dept. of Pathology, University of Michigan Medical School, Ann Arbor, Michigan (U.S.A.)

Zehnbauer B.A.
Dept. of Surgery, Anaesthesiology and Medicine, Washington University School of Medicine, St. Louis, Missouri (U.S.A.)

Abbreviations

APACHE, acute physiology and chronic health evaluation

ARDS, acute respiratory distress syndrome

AT, antithrombin

BPIP, bacterial permeability increasing protein

CARS, compensatory anti-inflammatory response syndrome

Cl_i, clearance of the I^{nth} component

CIS, cellular injury score

CLP, cecal ligation and puncture

COPD, chronic obstructive pulmonary disease

DIC, disseminated intravascular coagulation

DO_2, oxygen delivery

ECMO, extracorporeal membrane oxygenation

ESL-1, E-selectin ligand-1

FiO_2, % inspired oxygen

HGF, hepatocyte growth factor

Hsp, heat shock protein

ICAM-1, intercellular adhesion molecule-1

ICE, interleukin-1β converting enzyme

IL, interleukin

IL-1ra, interleukin-1 receptor antagonist

INH, isonicotinic acid hydrazide

ipH, intragastric pH

ISS, injury severity score

IVIG, intravenous immunoglobulin

MARS, mixed antagonistic response syndrome

MD, meningococcal disease

MODS, multiple organ dysfunction syndrome

MOF, multiple organ failure

NFκB, nuclear factor kappa B

NO, nitric oxide

O_2ER, oxygen extraction

$PaCO_2$, arterial carbon dioxide pressure

PAF, platelet activating factor

PAS, p-aminosalicylic acid

PCO_2, carbon dioxide pressure

PDH, pyruvate dehydrogenase

$PgCO_2$, gastric mucosal PCO_2

PGE1, prostaglandin

PIO_2, inspired PO_2

PMN, polymorphonuclear neutrophil

PVO_2, mixed venous PO_2

Q, perfusion

SAPS, simplified acute physiology score

SBITS, score-based immunoglobulin therapy of sepsis

SIRS, systemic inflammatory response syndrome

SOFA, sepsis-related organ failure assessment

sTNF-r, soluble tumor necrosis factor receptor

TNF, tumor necrosis factor

TSF, total splanchnic blood flow

TSH, thyroid stimulating hormone

VA, ventilation

$\dot{V}O_2$, oxygen consumption

Introduction

A.E. Baue

We welcome the readers to the Proceedings of the Seventh Annual Meeting of the Organ Failure Academy in Trieste, Italy. The Organ Failure Academy (OFA) was established by Professor Antonino Gullo in 1991 and the first meeting was held in 1992. I had the honor of being asked by Professor Gullo to serve as Honorary President of the OFA. The meetings of the OFA bring together distinguished scientists-clinicians from around the world to present and discuss their contributions to the care of the critically ill and injured.

This year the OFA meeting and these proceedings are dedicated to the memory of our good friend Roger Bone who died this year of metastatic renal cell carcinoma. A tribute to Dr. Bone is provided by Dr. Jean-Louis Vincent from Brussels who worked closely with Bone at many international meetings and publications in intensive care medicine.

We also note with sadness the sudden death of our friend and colleague Professor Gunther Schlag from Vienna.

This year the program and the proceedings were designed to review current concepts and raise questions about the importance and significance of various contributions. Our question this year is: What is real in the care of patients in the intensive care unit?

Questions have been raised about the importance and usefulness of the concepts of the systemic inflammatory response syndrome (SIRS) and the multiple organ dysfunction syndrome (MODS). Dr. Jean-Louis Vincent addresses this question in his presentation: "Shall we continue to talk about (or use) SIRS in the twenty-first century?". Dr. Vincent was one of the first senior-intensivists to raise questions about SIRS in his paper "Dear SIRS, I don't like you" [1]. Now he concludes that some will continue to use SIRS in the year 2000 because the idea is simple. However, he goes on to say that medicine is never simple and SIRS oversimplifies what is a very complex phenomenon so that playing with words does not help patients.

A few years ago dr. John Marshall and colleagues developed a scoring system for MODS [2]. With time and use of this system Dr. Marshall now addresses the question "Does a MODS score help the patient, the doctor or both?". Certainly it is true that, if treatment of MODS prevents the development of multiple organ failure (MOF), then that patient should have a better chance to survive. The classification, however, may or may not survive. There have been many classifications of MOF which are no longer used.

With injury, illness and sepsis, an inflammatory response is mounted. It is necessary for the patient but conventional wisdom tells us that overwhelming inflammation is a disaster for the individual and produces SIRS, MODS and MOF. Can we understand this process and this regulation? Can we ever hope to control or contain it and help the patient? Professor Peter Ward describes the endogenous control of the inflammatory process in the lung which raises the question as to whether we can support or expand these regulatory functions. Could they be worthwhile for therapy? Ward suggests that interventions to inhibit activation of NFκB may be useful. Dr. Stephen Lowry takes up the issue of whether we can ever hope to control the inflammatory process – reviewing the need for inflammation to heal and recover but also acknowledging that both too much and too little may be bad. Can we fool Mother Nature?

The basic biologic function of programmed cell death, or apoptosis, and how this activity is altered with sepsis and inflammation, provides a better understanding of the pathophysiology of illness. Dr. John Marshall and colleagues review the role of delayed neutrophil apoptosis in systemic inflammation and how this may contribute to remote organ dysfunction and failure. They describe restoration of normal expression of apoptosis in inflammatory neutrophils by IL-10 or by inhibition of ICE or Calpain. Dr. Timothy Buchman takes up the problem of "untimely" or delayed apoptosis and its place in modern patient care. Then, finally, they consider what we can do about it. Buchman believes that "therapeutics aimed at normalizing dysregulated cellular events may favorably affect clinical outcomes".

The failure of some, many or most clinical trials of so-called or potential "magic bullets" suggested that, if we could document the exact situation of a patient after injury, illness, operation or with sepsis, we could treat the patient more specifically or exactly by blocking or promoting some of the causes of the problem. Thus, great efforts were made to develop methods of early diagnosis of sepsis, of endotoxaemia, of molecular activation, and the phases of inflammation. Rapid endotoxin analyses in the emergency ward, rapid cultural techniques, methods to determine the presence of bacterial products in the bloodstream, cytokine analyses and other tests allow the early determination of these problems. The question to be considered is whether they will make any difference? Or is it just "so what?". Many cellular and intracellular events occur in sepsis. Measurement of Procalcitonin and IL-6 to predict or indicate the presence of sepsis are reviewed by Professor Konrad Reinhart who writes about "New and old markers of sepsis". The status of the early detection of endotoxins is reviewed by Dr. John Marshall. The question is – will it help our patients? Marshall believes that the chemiluminescent assay is a great help from their preliminary studies in identifying patients with Gram-negative infection.

Questions have been raised about animal research and whether or not it can contribute to the care of patients. I review for you the entire subject of clinical relevance of animal experimentation to human therapy and indicate where animal studies have contributed to patient care and also where they are of scientific interest but are probably unrelated to therapy in patients. We learn a lot about biology by animal experiments. Scientific studies in animals are critical and must continue. However, rats, mice, sheep, dogs and baboons are not people. In the past I have studied many potential therapeutic agents in animals which promised good results. Many or most of these never became clinically useful. Many animal studies end with a promissory note such as "These results (in 20 rats, mice, dogs, or sheep) have great potential clinical usefulness". I do not know why investigators in research do this but they do. There is no reason to give such promissory notes because most often these things do not work out clinically [3].

Specific organ or system support or other therapy to prevent MODS and MOF is reviewed in detail by a number of authors. Professor Ramsay and colleagues provide evidence for splanchnic perfusion being a critical factor in sepsis. They provide evidence for its having an important role in the pathophysiology of sepsis and organ failure.

Dr. De Backer reviews the methods of estimating the adequacy of splanchnic perfusion by intragastric pH and $PaCO_2$ monitoring in sepsis. Gastric $PaCO_2$ seems to be the wave of the future. De Backer also describes the effects of various agents and therapy upon gastric pHi and $PaCO_2$.

Professor Luciano Gattinoni and colleagues describe their observations in Milano of oxygen consumption and metabolism in trauma and sepsis and what might be done about it. Is it worthwhile to try to increase oxygen consumption, and when and in what patients? Gattinoni et al. provide evidence from their studies that maximizing oxygen transport does not necessarily reduce mortality.

Professor Pilz provides evidence for where and when intravenous immunoglobulins will help patients. Pilz indicates that, although no large control clinical trial of intravenous immunoglobulins (IVIG) has yet to document reduced mortality, there have been favorable responses in selected patients (e.g., early IVIG therapy decreases the severity of polyneuropathy in septic patients).

Dr. Michael Pinsky reviews biohumoral and immunomodulation factors in sepsis. He describes their work showing the circulating neutrophils in septic patients have an activated phenotype with CD11b and low L-selectin expression. Inflammation must represent a balance of intracellular NFκB activation and heat shock protein synthesis. Which patients then will benefit from augmenting or inhibiting neutrophil function remains to be determined.

Finally, I raise the question and review the experiences and evidence as to whether multiple agents, each of which reduces morbidity or improves some aspect of a patient's condition, can, if given together with a number of agents, reduce mortality. The problems of multiple-agent therapy are described. We should focus on specific diseases and problems such as trauma, peritonitis, pancreatitis, different causes of ARDS, etc. Treating all sick patients by nonspecific therapy for their disease have not worked.

Entirely new aspects of infection, sepsis, and organ failure in patients have now been discovered. One part of this is a genetic predisposition to human sepsis which is described by Dr. Timothy Buchman with Dr. Zehnbauer and Freeman. They describe genetic variations in TNF-α and TNF-β related to poor outcome in malaria and meningococcemia patients and IL-1 and its receptors may be related to susceptibility to infection. This emerging area of study is very exciting. Dr. Buchman has warned us about a therapy that improves some aspects of a patient but the patient dies anyway. This information greatly complicates clinical therapeutic trials – patients differ not only by age, sex, severity of illness and/or injury, but also genetically. Another difference is the exposure and immunologic memory of each individual [4]. There are great differences which influence therapy and response. I review these and other concepts in my paper on prevention and treatment of sepsis, MODS/MOF.

There is now a great revolution or evolution in science and particularly in biologic science. Previously we believed that there were actions and reactions. There were activators or mediators after injury or illness which were then controlled by anti-mediators. This is the homeostasis theory proposed by Walter Cannon. Now there is increasing evidence for a different form of biology. It is called integrative, or nonlinear, biology. It is part of CHAOS theory where influencing one factor alters the entire system. Thus, giving a monoclonal antibody to TNF to control the pro-inflammatory response alters not just TNF but the entire system. Professor Buchman comments on this in his writings. I provide evidence for this possibility in my review of "Injury, inflammation and sepsis – Is there a progression of endocrine and metabolic events during organ/system failures?".

This new concept in biology and physiology has been described and it will have a great impact on how we take care of patients and how we approach an inflammatory response. Stanley Schultz [5], in the Claude Bernard Lecture to the American Physiological Society, entitled "Homeostasis, Humpty Dumpty and integrative biology", described integrative biology. He stated that "in biology the parts are dynamic or plastic. They can change shape when they are brought together – that's what nonlinearity means". The shape of the whole cannot be predicted by knowing only the shapes of the separated parts. If you substitute function for shape, we can see that the function of the whole cannot be predicted by knowing only the functions of the separate parts. This seems to be where we are now in trying to determine pro-inflammatory mediators, anti-inflammatory mediators, and whatever.

Schultz goes on to say that molecular biology provides parts of a puzzle – "Putting them together is the problem". He reviewed Cannon's homeostasis concept and believed that homeodynamics would have been a jazzier and technically more correct expression. Tim Buchman stated: "If nested, nonlinear models are better representatives of human physiology than Cannon's collection of negative feedback, servomechanism, then therapy should be redirected toward transitions to a basal range – not therapeutically manipulating things such as cytokines or nitric oxide". Focusing on the phases of inflammation (pro-, anti-, etc.) would be Walter Cannon's approach. Blocking one mediator may change not only the effects of that mediator but may disturb other mediators in the entire system. As Buchman has also said, we are "prolonging lives far beyond the limited capacity of intrinsic physiologic responses" [6].

I referred to Lewis Thomas in my article on "Injury, inflammation, sepsis...". Lewis said: "The end result (of host defense) is not defense, it is an agitated committee-directed harum scarum effort to make war" [7]. Thus, we would like to think that our response to injury or illness is a highly organized, integrated and controlled biologic process. This seems to be true and can be described with modest or even moderate injury. However, with severe or overwhelming problems with injury and sepsis, it becomes, as Roger Bone described, "chaotic" [8]. Thomas' description should be of interest to us because he had great insight into the inflammatory process. The question is – Did Thomas see the beginning of nonlinearity in the new physiology or the new pathophysiology in human disease?

Sir Karl Popper, in his Medawar Lecture in 1986 to the Royal Society in London, said that "biology cannot be reduced to physics because biochemistry cannot be reduced to chemistry. Reductionism is not possible in biologic systems. An organism cannot be reduced to a series of systems" [9].

Weiss and Miller question: "How can mammals develop and maintain such a lethal defense system without ultimately harming themselves?" [10]. Many are studying this question. They state that "excessive or unrestricted use of this arsenal can result in injury to the host as can occur in autoimmune diseases, toxic shock syndrome and food poisoning". It is interesting that they do not mention or discuss the problems of overwhelming trauma and sepsis. The relationship of cytokines and inflammatory cells can be: 1) an interaction which is successful in host defense; 2) unsuccessful in immune deficiency problems; 3) inappropriate in autoimmunity and allergy; 4) perhaps inappropriate also with severe illness and injury.

In my chapter on prevention and treatment of sepsis, I review two ideas which complicate our thinking about our sick patients. One I call "harbingers of doom" or critical events which predict disaster. There are many examples of this and the question is – Are they mediators (contributing to the disaster) or just markers of trouble? The other idea is about "biologic conundrums" or puzzles. There are also many examples of this where an agent, a mediator causes trouble injecting TNF into animals or patients but, in other circumstances, that mediator is required for survival. Can we ever hope to understand all of these complexities?

I also review the concept that curing a disease, healing an injury or reducing mortality requires specific therapy for the cause of that problem. Thus, we must become "splinters, not lumpers".

Our host Professors Berlot and Gullo contribute to this book a review of what is wrong and what is right about studies in progress in sepsis and MODS. They discuss the gap between experimental findings and clinical results and new information which could change some of the previous negative trials of the so-called "magic bullets" [11]. Better results could be possible by better agents (anti-endotoxins), different time frames, different endpoints, and more patients enrolled.

We hope that the information provided for you in the chapters of this book will help you to better care for your patients. The question has been raised as to whether death or mortality is the best endpoint of clinical trials of potentially better therapy. However, if one of our treatments improves the patient to some extent, but the patient dies anyway, what is gained? I review this dilemma in the chapter on "The potential of multiple therapeutic agents".

We come, then, to a summary of what this is all about. Although we must strive to learn more about our patients and the problems of sepsis and inflammation, we must strive to prevent injury, sepsis, SIRS, MODS and MOF. Once they occur, we will do our best, but frequently it is too late.

The biologic response to injury serves to maintain the viability of the organism under adverse circumstances. Understanding of this response, its variations and its pathologic distortions, allow a physician to treat injured patients properly. The organism copes with modest injury by maintaining perfusion of vital organs, mobilizing body water and altering metabolism to heal the injury, a response essential for survival. An inflammatory response is necessary. When the injury is overwhelming, however, the response also becomes overwhelming and potentially destructive. The consequences may include many problems for the patient.

I hope we have stimulated you to help attack some of these problems in patient care. Advances come from observations, ideas, clinical trials and refusing to accept dogma without proof. All of you can participate in, and contribute to, such progress. Our patients need all of the help we can give them.

References

1. Vincent JL (1997) Dear SIRS, I'm sorry to say I don't like you. Crit Care Med 25:372-374
2. Marshall JC, Cook DA, Sibbald W et al (1992) The Multiple Organ Dysfunction (MOD) score: a reliable descriptor of a complex clinical outcome. Crit Care Med 20:580-587
3. Baue AE (1998) The promissory note in scientific research. Am J Surg 175:2-3
4. Bennett-Guerrero E, Ayuso L, Hamilton-Davis et al (1997) Relationship of preoperative anti-endotoxin core antibodies and adverse outcomes following cardiac surgery. JAMA 277: 646-650
5. Schultz S (1996) Homeostasis, Humpty Dumpty and integrative biology. News Physiol Sci 11:238-246
6. Buchman T (1996) Physiologic stability and physiologic state. J Trauma 41:599-605
7. Thomas L (1970) Adaptive aspects of inflammation. Symposium of the Int Inflammation Club, Kalamazoo, Michigan; UpJohn Co
8. Bone RC (1996) Sir Isaac Newton, Sepsis, SIRS and CARS. Crit Care Med 24:1125-1138
9. Popper K (1986) The Medawar Lecture on Biology. Proc Royal Soc, London
10. Weiss A, Miller LJ (1998) Halting the march of the immune defenses. Science 280:179
11. Baue AE (1997) MOF, MODS, SIRS - Why no magic bullets? Arch Surg 132:1-5

BASIC PATHOPHYSIOLOGY MECHANICS

Inflammation: How Much Is Too Much and Can It Be Controlled?

V. Rumalla, S.F. Lowry

The human immune response to infection includes an orchestration of various specific and non-specific soluble factors and cellular elements. The appropriate response leads to efficient control of infection or repair of injury; but when this response is too little or too much it may result in a completely different outcome. An attenuated immune defense leads to poor healing and prolonged infection. By contrast, an exaggerated response may result in shock and multi-system organ failure [1-3]. It is a balanced and regulated immune cascade which most predictably leads to recovery. Among the areas of most intense current interest is an understanding of the mechanics which promote such activation and control of the immune response to inflammation.

Many of the same pro-inflammatory mediators necessary for wound healing and host defense have also been implicated in the systemic inflammatory response syndrome (SIRS). The precipitating causes of SIRS can be sufficiently diverse; including infection, trauma, surgery, and pancreatitis that describing any specific mechanism or developing a unified therapeutic intervention becomes difficult [4]. Thus, the question arises as to how the immune response might be modulated to achieve the desired effect of recovery under seemingly disparate conditions.

The pro-inflammatory cytokines TNF and IL-1 are known to be important in initiating the inflammatory response. In vitro and pre-clinical studies used to blunt and block these cytokines have led to dramatic attenuation of many consequences of the immune response. At the same time, studies also suggest that at points subsequent to severe injury or haemorrhage, in fact, cytokine production capacity may be diminished [5-7]. Hence, blunting the immune response under these circumstances may be detrimental. To answer the above question, we will examine the pro-inflammatory state and the body's natural counter-regulatory mechanisms which are elucidated as part of the initial immune response to injury. Secondly, a closer look at studies and clinical trials designed to blunt pro-inflammatory cytokines will serve to outline the potential utility as well as problems associated with various "anti"-inflammatory measures.

Pro-inflammatory cytokines

Tumor necrosis factor

Tumor necrosis factor (TNF) is secreted primarily by the macrophage-monocyte line of cells and it has quite diverse effects. TNF is important in initiating the immune cascade after the body is stressed by injury or bacteria. A variety of stimuli including parasites, tumors, and endotoxin stimulate cells to produce TNF [8-10]. TNF is also involved in the recruitment and maturation of the cellular component of inflammation. This is manifested by the increased neutrophil release from the bone marrow, margination, and cytotoxicity [11]. In addition, TNF is essential in the upregulation of cell surface adhesion molecules which are crucial during the cell to endothelium interface which is necessary for neutrophil chemotaxis [12, 13]. It is well known from the wound healing literature that tissue levels of TNF have important paracrine effects in initiating proper and expedient healing [14, 15]. These local effects include haemostasis, increased vascular permeability, increased vascular proliferation, and collagen synthesis [12]. Finally, TNF has many metabolic effects including a contribution toward promoting the supply of nutrient substrates, acute phase protein production, and wound healing [11]. A diminished TNF response has been associated with poor outcomes in inflammatory states [2, 3].

By contrast, excessive production of TNF may also lead to deleterious consequences, being implicated in multi-system organ failure and associated with increased morbidity and mortality [16-20]. The deleterious effects of TNF include circulatory collapse, hypotension, and damage to solid organs [10, 21, 22]. This effect is clearly multidimensional. It includes the procoagulant effects of TNF which favor thrombosis of the microcirculation, increased vascular permeability and myocardial depression, as well as the recruitment and activation of various immune cells [23, 24]. These immune cells lead to increased tissue damage by the production of reactive metabolites, proteolytic enzymes, and arachidonic acid metabolites [25, 26].

Interleukin 1

Interleukin 1 (IL-1) shares many properties of TNF although with less capacity to produce shock. IL-1 is also produced by cells of the monocyte-macrophage line. Similar to TNF, IL-1 activates neutrophils, upregulates adhesion molecules, and promotes chemotaxis [11]. IL-1 also effects coagulation and tends to favor thrombosis while TNF still retains potent anti-coagulant properties [23, 27-29]. In addition, IL-1 promotes other cells like endothelial cells to secrete pro-inflammatory cytokines [30]. In the central nervous system, IL-1 appears to elicit a febrile response and is important in the regulation of the pituitary counter-regulatory hormone axis [31, 32]. Like TNF, many of the effects of IL-1 are important in wound healing and the activity of IL-1 response may be essential to longer term host defense [2]. While some studies implicate increased IL-1 levels with sepsis, cachexia, and chronic disease [33-37], others show that lower levels of circulating IL-1 are associated with greater mortality in burn patients [38, 39] and may contribute to the immune anergy seen in trauma patients [40].

Interleukin 6

IL-6 is a very pleuri-potent cytokine with a large variety of functions. IL-6's most important functions include stem cell growth, B and T lymphocyte activation, and the regulation of the hepatic acute phase protein response [41-45]. These acute phase proteins are essential in the host's immune, coagulation, and metabolic response. IL-6 is synthesized by many cells in the body, but like the other pro-inflammatory cytokines, the cells of the macrophage and monocyte line appear to be very important. IL-6 is released in response to multiple stimuli, TNF, IL-1, and endotoxin being potent agonists [46, 47]. In vivo, circulating levels of IL-6 are increased during both acute bacteraemia and chronic disease states in humans. Unlike IL-1 and TNF, circulating levels of IL-6 are routinely detected in most states associated with inflammation [2, 48-50]. In fact, studies show that IL-6 plasma levels were higher in nonsurvivors vs. survivors of burns, pancreatitis, and sepsis [51]. The nearly uniform presence of soluble IL-6 in the circulation during disease states makes it an attractive marker for outcomes but, to date, a lack of uniform standards for IL-6 detection has precluded large scale analysis of IL-6 as a marker for disease severity.

Cytokine therapy

Given the role of cytokines in inflammation and multi-system organ failure, investigators have sought to attenuate the inflammatory response through various immunomodulatory strategies. Data suggested that effective control of excessive pro-inflammatory cytokines might benefit patients with severe infection or inflammation. With the rapid development of several anti-cytokine agents, broad ranging pre-clinical and clinical studies sought to address this concept.

Anti-TNF antibodies

TNF blockade offers an interesting mean to reduce the detrimental effects of the cytokine. Prior studies using specific anti-TNF antibodies during gram negative sepsis have shown some improvement in haemodynamics and survival, but the results are not all optimistic [52-56]. Specifically, the timing of administration of such therapy appears essential to improve outcomes. Studies conducted where anti-TNF antibody was given prior to bacterial or endotoxin challenge were more effective in preventing circulatory collapse and shock. This benefit of pre-treatment directly relates to the kinetics of TNF production, where the peak appearance of bioactive protein occurs within ninety minutes of an endotoxin challenge and drops to pre-challenge levels within three hours [9]. Thus any initial TNF influences are erected early in the inflammatory process. The effect of anti-TNF therapy in experimental sepsis models includes a decrease in vascular congestion, haemorrhage, leukocyte adhesion, and circulatory collapse [55]. Specifically, anti-TNF therapy has been shown to improve left ventricular stroke volume [57]. On the contrary, some investigators have failed to show any beneficial effect of anti-TNF therapy and some even show decreased survival, especially in chronic models of infection/inflammation where low levels of TNF activity are neutralized [58-60]. Similarly, virtually all clinical trials with anti-TNF antibodies have failed to show decreased mortality [61, 62].

Soluble TNF receptors

Unlike anti-TNF monoclonal antibodies, soluble TNF receptors (sTNF-r) are naturally occurring soluble forms of the two TNF receptors found on cells. These soluble proteins bind with the same relative affinity to circulating TNF as do the cell associated forms [63-66]. An inverse relationship between cell associated and soluble receptor in a sepsis model illustrates that soluble receptors represent shed receptor from the cell. This process of shedding receptors may confer some protection to the cell from the effect of circulating TNF. Soluble TNF-r has been identified in the blood and urine of both acutely septic patients as well as chronic disease states [67, 68]. Following the administration of LPS, sTNF-r is detected in the blood contemporaneously with the ligand and persists for several hours beyond the time of detectable TNF levels [69]. Studies in our own lab, and others, have shown that higher circulating levels of sTNF-r were found in survivors over non-survivors of sepsis [70].

Recombinant forms of TNF receptors binding proteins have been developed and used in pre-clinical trials [71, 72]. Administration of these proteins has been shown to have a protective effect during injury but had to be given in very large 300x molar excess to achieve this effect [11]. This is due in part to the very low concentration of TNF required to activate the cell. Also, studies show that in patients with severe sepsis, a p55 TNF-r fusion protein was associated with a 36% decrease in overall mortality compared to placebo [73]. However, not all data demonstrate conclusive evidence that an overall decrease in mortality is achieved. Van Zee et al. showed in primate models that though a p55 soluble receptor yielded initial improvement in cardiac haemodynamics, this improvement deteriorated and the overall mortality was not decreased [74]. The deterioration in this study was accompanied by a rise in TNF bioactivity in the plasma and the authors expounded that this effect may have been secondary to receptor-ligand dissolution. Similarly, studies by Fisher et al. showed that p75 TNF-r fusion protein did not reduce overall mortality and at higher doses was even associated with greater mortality [75].

IL-1 receptor antagonist

Like TNF, IL-1 also has a naturally occurring soluble receptor antagonist, IL-1ra. IL-1ra binds with high affinity to either IL-1 receptors without any known agonist activity [76] and is synthesized by many cell lines [77-79]. IL-1ra is released in response to a variety of stimuli including IL-1, IL-6 [80], and endotoxin administration in both primate and human models [81]. In addition, clinical studies have shown similar appearance in the circulation in trauma, infection, chronic disease [82], and septic shock [83]. However, in sepsis the endogenous production of IL-1ra may be insufficient to neutralize the effects of IL-1 [84, 85]. Slotman et al. showed that IL-1ra infusion in a human sepsis trial reduced the synthesis of various eicosanoids and IL-6 production while plasma IL-1 levels rose [86]. In addition, non-steroidal anti-inflammatory drugs have been recently shown to increase IL-1ra without increasing IL-1 [87]. However, not all studies echo optimism. In neonatal sepsis inadequate IL-1ra production did not correlate with increased mortality [88] and in fact higher levels were found in non-survivors vs. survivors of adult burn-related sepsis [89].

A recombinant form of the protein has been cloned and used extensively in experimental models. Shito et al. showed that pre-treatment with IL-1ra reduced histologic damage to liver parenchyma in a hepatic ischaemia reperfusion model in mice [90]. Other in vitro and primate studies have shown that the presumed effects of IL-1 can be blocked by the administration of IL-1ra, but only when given at a 100-1000x molar excess of predicted IL-1 concentration [11]. On the contrary, studies in mice abscesses showed no clinical improvement with IL-1ra administration and that higher doses was associated with increased morbidity [91]. In addition, recently terminated clinical trials in septic patients with IL-1ra showed no decreased mortality compared to controls [92]. Though IL-1ra has been shown to block the effect of IL-1, very low levels of active IL-1 are needed to produce its biological effect making adequate receptor blockade a difficult therapeutic intervention. New isoforms of the receptor antagonist have been cloned and await clinical trials [93].

Interleukin 10

IL-10 is a potent anti-inflammatory cytokine. It mediates this effect through the inhibition of gene expression and synthesis of the major pro-inflammatory cytokines TNF, IL-1, and IL-6 [85, 94]. In addition, IL-10 has been shown to increase IL-1ra synthesis [95]. Plasma levels of IL-10 have been detected in the circulation of patients with sepsis and animals injected with LPS [83, 96, 97]. In addition, it is elevated in critically ill patients versus controls [98]. In vitro studies have shown that IL-10 administration suppresses endotoxin induced TNF synthesis while IL-10 neutralization led to increased TNF production [99]. More importantly, several studies show that exogenously administered IL-10 or gene transfer in LPS injected mice conferred protection and was associated with a decreased mortality [100, 101].

Endocrine response

Central to the body's counter-regulatory immune mechanism is the endocrine response. The hypothalamic-pituitary-adrenal axis is essential to most homeostatic mechanisms in the body. Particularly both glucocorticoids and catecholamines play an important role in the immune system. It is known that glucocorticoids have a prominent effect on the production and effect of pro-inflammatory cytokines. Animal studies clearly show that glucocorticoid administration blunts the production IL-1, TNF, and IL-6 at both the transcriptional and translational level [102-106]. As for IL-6, there appears to be an additional effect of decreased production of acute phase proteins. Inflammation in general, especially circulating TNF and IL-1, appears to have a positive feedback response on the macro-endocrine system [107]. In vitro studies using TNF and IL-1 on hypothalamic and pituitary cells led to the increased synthesis of corticotropin releasing factor and adrenocorticotropic hormone [108-111]. Interestingly, this effect can be blunted by the administration of exogenous glucocorticoids [112]. In addition, pro-inflammatory cytokine blockade itself leads to diminished glucocorticoid response during severe bacteraemia. However, in less severe states of infection cytokine blockade did not yield similar response [113].

Many experimental applications of glucocorticoids have been attempted. Human experiments have shown that cortisol administration reduces the production of TNF during endotoxaemia [114]. Additional animal studies demonstrate that glucocorticoids are protective in septic shock [11]. Unfortunately not all results have been encouraging. This is in part due to the fact that glucocorticoid mediated TNF suppression may be reversed or overcome by other cytokines like interferon γ [104]. Additionally, dexamethasone was shown to antagonize the release of IL-1ra and IL-10 both crucial anti-inflammatory cytokines during in vitro studies [115, 116]. In fact, a recently published met-analysis of nine glucocorticoid therapy clinical trials in septic patients showed no decrease in mortality while several of the individual studies themselves showed increased mortality [117].

Like corticosteroids, catecholamines appear to have potent inflammatory effects [118]. For example, norepinephrine has been shown to directly reduce TNF and IL-6 in whole blood models [119]. In addition, the local production of cathecholamines has been shown to increase corticosterone production [113]. Finally, epinephrine infusion does reduce TNF appearance after endotoxin administration in human studies [120].

Conclusion

There appears to be no panacea for sepsis and SIRS at this time. Central to our failure at therapeutic interventions is most likely our incomplete understanding of the inflammatory process itself. As new cytokines are discovered and new immune mechanisms elucidated, the picture may become clearer. Several comments can be made from our current understanding of inflammation. First, acute inflammation is necessary for host defense, repair, and homeostasis. Of importance, pro-inflammatory cytokines are essential in this process especially locally in injured or damaged tissues. However, when produced in excess, these same cytokines tend to spill into the circulation and can have profound deleterious systemic effects. It is also known that the immune system possesses many inherent anti-inflammatory mechanisms. Teleologically, it appears that the body anticipates or has learned that profound or even excess inflammation may be in part necessary to achieve the outcome of recovery from injury. Many studies support this line of thought.

However, an excess anti-inflammatory response may also lead to poor outcomes. Roger Bone, along with others, has addressed the theory and coined the term compensatory anti-inflammatory response syndrome (CARS) [3]. This anti-inflammatory response may lead to a state of immunosuppression which makes the host more susceptible to infection. Several correlations with CARS and poor outcomes in burns, trauma, and pancreatitis have been made [3, 121].

Thus, it makes sense that controlling the inflammatory response is more important than preventing it. The first goal of therapy appears to allow an adequate host defense at that sites of injury while preventing high systemic levels of pro-inflammatory mediators. The inflammatory response has been initiated well before patients most present for medical attention or before a change in clinical state has been noticed.

However, this brings us to our next question – when is the right time to implement therapy? If we wait till the clinical signs of sepsis or severe inflammation appear, studies have shown that anti-inflammatory therapies may improve some of these septic parameters, but no overall decrease in mortality is uniformly achieved. At the same time, when these interventions are given in excess, our review points to studies which show similarly poor outcomes.

Once the decision to institute anti-inflammatory therapy is made, the final question lies in selecting the type of intervention. Our review of the pro- and anti-inflammatory immune cascade elucidated several places for therapeutic intervention, as well as the data from in vitro and in vivo clinical trials with various

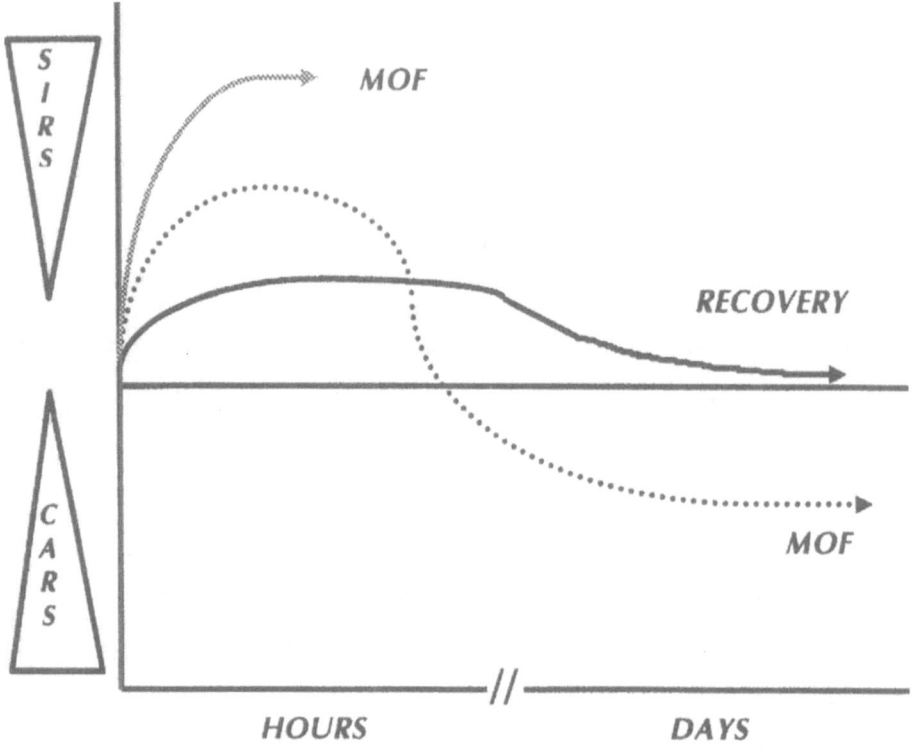

Fig. 1. Schematic representation of the acute systemic inflammatory response to an injurious event that exceeds compensatory influences may rapidly lead to tissue injury, multiple organ failure (MOF), and death (solid gray line). A lesser inflammatory response followed by overcompensation by compensatory anti-inflammatory response (CARS) mechanisms may render an immunosuppressed state that is also detrimental to the host (interrupted line). Controlled injury elicits the necessary inflammatory mediators, but is followed by timely return to homeostasis. (Modified from [81])

agents. Again, no clearly superior therapy was noted, but the results do support cautious optimism. The failure of clinical trials to show large improvement in outcomes lies in part in patient selection and the number of subjects.

In the end, our current understanding of inflammation leads us to believe that in part it must be supported like other metabolic functions in the body such as nutrition and hydration. However, careful vigilance must be maintained. Thus, further study to help identify the markers and signs that predict the clinical appearance of sepsis and multi-system organ failure, as well as larger clinical trials, may be the most crucial step in treating this complex condition.

References

1. Davies MG, Hagen PO(1997) Systemic inflammatory response syndrome. Br J Surg 84:920
2. Bone RC (1996) Toward a theory regarding the pathogenesis of the systemic inflammatory response syndrome. What we do and do not know about cytokine regulation. Crit Care Med 24:163
3. Bone RC (1996) Immunologic dissonance: a continuing evolution in our understanding of the systemic inflammatory response and the multiple organ dysfunction syndrome. Ann Intern Med 125:680
4. Nystrom PO (1998) The systemic inflammatory response syndrome. J Antimicrob Chemother 41:A1
5. Schmand JF, Ayala A, Morrison MH, Chaudry IH (1995) Effects of hydroxyethyl starch after trauma hemorragic shock: restoration of macrophage integrity and prevention of increased circulating interleukin-6. Crit Care Med 23:806
6. Chaudry IH, Ayala A, Ertel W, Stephan RN (1990) Hemorrhage and resuscitation: immunological aspects. Am J Physiol 259:R663
7. Meldrum DR, Ayala A, Perrin MM et al (1991) Diltiazem restores IL-2, IL-3, IL-6, and IFN-gamma synthesis and decreased host susceptibility to sepsis following hemorrage. J Surg Res 51:158
8. Kunkel SL, Remick DG, Strieter RM, Larrick JW (1989) Mechanisms that regulate the production and effects of tumor necrosis factor alpha. Crit Rev Immunol 9:93
9. Michie HR, Manogue KR, Spriggs DR et al (1988) Detection of circulating tumor necrosis factor after endotoxin administration. N Engl J Med 318:3972
10. Bauss F, Droge W, Mannel DN (1988) Tumor necrosis factor mediates endotoxic effects in mice. Infect Immun 55:1622
11. Fong Y, Lowry SF (1996) Cytokines and the cellular response to injury and infection. Scientific American, vol II: Care in the ICU
12. Greenfield LJ, Mulholland MW, Oldham KT, Zelenock GB, and Lillemore KD (eds) (1997) Surgery: Scientific principles and practice, 2nd edn. Lippincott-Raven, Philadelphia
13. Moser R, Schleiffenbaum B, Groscurth P et al (1989) Interleukin 1 and tumor necrosis factor stimulate human vascular endothelial cells to promote transendothelial neutrophil passage. J Clin Invest 83:444
14. Clark RAF (1993) Basics of cutaneous wound repair. J Dermatol Surg Oncol 19:693
15. Salomon GD, Kasid A, Cromack DT et al (1991) The local effects of cachectin/tumor necrosis factor on wound healing. Ann Surg 214:175
16. Girardin E, Grau GE, Dayer JM et al (1988) Tumor necrosis factor and interleukin 1 in the serum of children with severe infectious purpura. N Engl J Med 319:397
17. Marks JD, Marks CB, Luce JM et al (1990) Plama tumor necrosis factor in patients with septic shock: mortality rate, incidence of adult respiratory distress syndrome. Am Rev Respir Dis 141:94
18. Shalaby MR, Halgunset J, Haugen OA et al (1991) Cytokine-associated tissue injury and lethality in mice: a comparative study. Clin Immunol Immunopathol 61:69
19. Waage A, Halstensen A, Espevik T (1987) Association between tumor necrosis factor in serum and fatal outcome in patients with meningococcal disease. Lancet 1:355
20. Mustafa MM, Lebel MH, Ramilo O et al (1989) Correlation of interleukin 1 beta and cachectin concentrations in cerebrospinal fluid and outcome from bacterial menigitis. J Pediatr 115:208
21. Tracey KJ, Beutler B, Lowry SF et al (1986) Shock and tissue injury induced by recombinant human cachectin. Science 234:470
22. Remick DJ, Kunkel RG, Larrick JW, Kunkel SL (1987) Acute in vivo effects of human recombinant tumor necrosis factor. Lab Invest 56:583
23. Bevilacqua MP, Pober JS, Majeau GR et al (1986) Recombinant tumor necrosis factor induces procoagulant activity in cultured human vascular endothelium: characterization and comparison with the actions of interleukin 1. Proc Natl Acad Sci USA 83:4533

24. Nawroth PP, Stern DM (1986) Modulation of endothelial cell hemostatic properties by tumor necrosis factor. J Exp Med 163:740
25. Strieter RM, Lynch III JP, Basha MA et al (1990) Host responses in mediating sepsis and the adult respiratory distress syndrome. Semin Respir Infect 5:233
26. Tracey KJ, Lowry SF, Cerami A (1988) Cachectin/TNF-alpha in the septic shock and septic adult respiratory distress syndrome. Am Rev Respir Dis 138:1377
27. Nachman RL, Hajjar KA, Siverstein RL, Dinarello CA (1986) Interleukin 1 induces endothelial cell synthesis of plasminogen activator inhibitor. J Exp Med 163:1595
28. Gramse M, Brevario F, Pintucci G et al (1986) Enhancement by interleukin 1 of plasminogen activator inhibitor activity in cultured human endothelial cells. Biochem Biophys Res Commun 139:720
29. Nawroth PP, Handley DA, Esmon CT et al (1986) Interleukin 1 induces endothelial cell procoagulant while suppressing cell surface anticoagulant activity. Proc Natl Acad USA 83:3460
30. Loppnow H, Bil R, Hirt S et al (1998) Platelet derived interleukin 1 induces cytokine production, but not proliferation of human vascular smooth muscle cells. Blood 91:134
31. Van Dam AM, Poole S, Schulzberg M et al (1998) Effects of peripheral administration of LPS on the expression of immunoreactive interleukin-1 alpha, beta, and receptor antagonist in rat brain. Ann NY Acad Sci 840:128
32. Lang CH, Fan J, Wogner MM et al (1998) Role of central IL-1 in regulating peripheral IGF-1 during endotoxemia and sepsis. Am J Physiol 274: R956
33. Fischer E, Marano MA, Van Zee KJ et al (1992) Interleukin 1 receptor blockade improves survival and hemodynamic performance in Escherichia coli septic shock, but fails to alter host response to sublethal endotoxinemia. J Clin Invest 89:1551
34. Ohlsson K, Bjork P, Bergenfeldt M et al (1990) Interleukin 1 receptor antagonist reduces mortality from endotoxin shock. Nature 346:550
35. Alexander HR, Doherty GM, Buresh CM et al (1991) A recombinant human receptor antagonist interleukin 1 improves survival after lethal endotoxemia in mice. J Exp Med 173:1029
36. Barriere SL, Lowry SF (1995) An overview of mortality risk prediction in sepsis. Crit Care Med 23:376
37. Fong YM, Moldawer LL, Marano MA et al (1989) Cachectin/TNF or IL-1 alpha induces cachexia with redistribution of body proteins. Am J Physiol 256:R659
38. Cannon JG, Friedberg JS, Gelfand JA et al (1992) Circulating interleukin 1B and tumor necrosis concentrations after burn injury in humans. Crit Care Med 20:1414
39. Mills CD, Caldwell MD, Gann DS (1989) Evidence of plasma-mediated "window" of immunodeficiency in rats following trauma. J Clin Immunol 9:139
40. Browder W, Williams D, Pretus H et al (1990) Beneficial effect of enhanced macrophage function in the trauma patient. Ann Surg 211:605
41. Akira S, Hirano T, Taga T, Kishimoto T (1990) Biology of multifunctional cytokines: IL-6 and related molecules (IL-1, and TNF). FASEB J 4:2860
42. Kopf M, Baumann H, Freer G et al (1994) Impaired immune and acute phase responses in interleukin 6 deficient mice. Nature 368:339
43. Castell JV, Gomez-Lechon M, David M et al (1989) Interleukin-6 is the major regulator of acute phase response protein synthesis in adult human hepatocytes. FEBS 242:237
44. Gauldie J, Baumann H (1991) Cytokines and acute phase protein expression. In: Kimball EH (ed) Cytokines in inflammation. Telford Press, Toronto
45. Heinrich PC, Castell JV, Andus T (1990) Interleukin 6 and acute phase response. Biochem J 265:621
46. Fong Y, Moldawer LL, Marano M et al (1989) Endotoxemia elicits increased circulating b-IFN/IL-6 in man. J Immunol 142:2321
47. Hack CE, DeGroot ER, Felt-Bersma RJF et al (1989) Increased plama levels of interleukin 6 in sepsis. Blood 74:1704
48. Castell JV, Gomez-Lechon M, David M et al (1989) Interleukin-6 is the major regulator of acute phase response protein synthesis in adult human hepatocytes. FEBS 242:237

49. Gauldie J, Northermann W, Fey GH (1990) IL-6 function as an endocrine hormone in inflammation: Hepatocytes undergoing acute phase protein response require exogenous IL-6. J Immunol 144:3804
50. Calandra T, Gerain J, Heumann D et al (1991) High circulating levels of IL-6 in patients with septic shock: evolution during sepsis, prognostic value and interplay with other cytokines. Am J Med 91:23
51. Frieling JT, van Deuren M, Wijdenes J et al (1995) Circulating interleukin 6 receptor in patients with sepsis syndrome. J Infect Dis 17:469
52. Abraham E (1998) Cytokine modifiers: pipe dream or reality? Chest 113[Suppl 3]:224S
53. Tracey KJ, Yuman F, Hesse DG et al (1987) Anti-cachectin/TNF monoclonal antibodies prevent septic shock during letal bacteremia. Nature 330:662
54. Fong Y, Atracey KJ, Moldawer LL et al (1989) Antibodies to cachectin/tumor necrosis factor reduces interleukin 1 beta and interleukin 6 appearance during lethal bacteremia. J Exp Med 170:1627
55. Hinshaw LB, Emerson TE, Taylor FB et al (1992) Lethal Staphylococcus Aureus-induced shock in primates: prevention of death with anti-TNF antibody. J Trauma 33:568
56. Mohler K, Torrance D, Smith C et al (1993) Soluble tumor necrosis factor receptors are effective therapeutic agents in lethal endotoxemia and function simultaneously as both carriers and TNF antagonists. J Immunol 151:1548
57. Vincent JL, Bakker J, Marecaux G et al (1992) Administration of anti-TNF antibody improves left ventricular function in septic shock patients. Chest 101:810
58. Eskandri MK, Bolgos G, Miller C et al (1992) Anti-tumor necrosis antibody therapy fails to prevent lethality after cecal ligation and puncture or endotoxinemia. J Immunol 148:2724
59. Wayte J, Silva A, Krausz T, Cohen J (1993) Observations on the role of tumor necrosis factor in a murine model of shock due to Streptococcus Pyogenes. Crit Care Med 21:1207
60. Sawyer RG, Adams RB, May AK et al (1993) Anti-tumor necrosis factor antibody reduces mortality in the presence of antibiotic. Arch Surg 128:173
61. Reinhart K, Wiegand-Lohnert C, Grimminger F (1996) Assessment of the safety and efficacy of the monoclonal anti-tumor necrosis factor monoclonal antibody fragment, MAK 195, in patients with sepsis and septic shock: A multicenter, randomized, placebo-controlled, dose ranging study. Crit Care Med 24:733
62. Dhainaut JFA, Vincent JL, Richard C (1995) CDP571, a humanized antibody to human necrosis factor alpha: Safety, pharmacokinetics, immune response, and influence of the antibody on the cytokine concentrations in patients with septic shock. Crit Care Med 23:1461
63. Ryffel B, Mihatsch MJ (1993) TNF receptor distribution in human tissues. Int Rev Exp Pathol 34:149
64. Tartaglia LA, Goeddel DV (1992) Tumor necrosis factor receptor signaling: a dominant negative mutation suppresses the activation of 55 kDA tumor necrosis factor receptor. J Biol Chem 267:4304
65. Tartaglia LA, Pennica D, Goeddel DV (1993) Ligand passing: the 75 kDa tumor necrosis factor receptor recruits TNF signaling by the p55 TNF receptor. J Biol Chem 25:18542
66. Loetscer H, Stueber D, Banner D et al (1993) Human tumor necrosis factor alpha mutants with exclusive specificity for the 55 kd or 75 kd TNF receptors. J Biol Chem 268:26350
67. Engelman H, Aderka A, Rubinstein M et al (1989) A tumor necrosis factor binding protein purified to homogeneity from human urine protects from tumor necrosis factor toxicity. J Biol Chem 20:11974
68. Heilig B, Fiehn C, Brockhaus M et al (1993) Evaluation of soluble tumor necrosis factor receptor antibodies in patients with systemic lupus erythematosus, progressive systemic sclerosis, and mixed connective tissue disease. J Clin Immunol 13:321
69. Neilson D, Kavanagh JP, Rao PN (1996) Kinetics of circulating TNF alpha and TNF soluble receptors following surgery in a clinical model of sepsis. Cytokine 8:938
70. Calvano SE, van der Poole T, Coyle SM et al (1996) Monocyte tumor necrosis factor levels as a predictor of risk in human sepsis. Arch Surg 131:434

71. Read RC (1998) Experimental therapies for sepsis directed against tumor necrosis factor. J Antimicrob Chemother 41:65
72. Bertini R, Delgado R, Faggioni R et al (1993) Urinary TNF-binding protein protects mice against the lethal effect of TNF and endotoxin shock. Eur Cytokine Network 4:39
73. Abraham E, Glauser MP, Butler T et al (1997) p55 Tumor necrosis factor fusion protein in the treatment of patients with severe sepsis and septic shock. A randomized controlled multicenter trial. Ro 45-2081 Study Group. JAMA 277:1531
74. Van Zee KJ, Kohno T, Fischer E et al (1992) Tumor necrosis factor soluble receptors circulate during experimental and clinical inflammation and can protect against excessive tumor necrosis factor alpha in vitro and in vivo. Proc Natl Acad Sci USA 89:4845
75. Fisher CJ Jr, Agosti JM, Opal SM et al (1996) Treatment of septic shock with the tumor necrosis factor receptor: Fc fusion protein. The Soluble TNF Receptor Sepsis Study Group. N Engl J Med 334:1697
76. Shimauchi H, Takayama S, Imai-Tanaka T, Okada H (1998) Balance of interleukin-1 beta and interleukin-1 receptor antagonist in human periapical lesions. J Endod 24:116
77. Matsukawa A, Fukumoto T, Maeda T et al (1997) Detection and characterization of Il-1 receptor antagonist in tissues from healthy rabbits: Il-1 receptor antagonist is probably involved in health. Cytokine 9:307
78. Eisenberg SP, Evans RJ, Arend WP et al (1990) Primary structure and functional expression from complementary DNA of human interleukin-1 receptor antagonist. Nature 343:341
79. Dripps DJ, Brandhuber BJ, Thompson RC, Eisenberg SP (1991) Interleukin 1 (IL-1) receptor antagonist binds to the 80-kDa IL-1 receptor but does not initiate IL-1 signal transduction. J Biol Chem 16:10331
80. Gabay C, Smith MF, Eidlen D, Arend WP (1997) Interleukin-1 receptor antagonist is an acute phase protein. J Clin Invest 99:2813
81. Guirao X, Lowry S (1996) Biologic control of injury and inflammation: much more than too little or too late. World J Surg 20:437
82. Fukomoto T, Matsukawa A, Ohkawara S et al (1996) Administration of neutralizing antibody against rabbit IL-1 receptor antagonist exacerbates lipopolysaccharide induced arthritis in rabbits. Inflamm Res 45:479
83. Kasai T, Inada K, Takakuwa Y et al (1997) Anti-inflammatory cytokine levels in patients with septic shock. Res Commun Mol Pathol Phamacol 98:34
84. Dinarello CA, Wolff SM (1993) The role of IL-1 in disease. N Engl J Med 328:106
85. Fischer E, Van Zee KJ, Marano M et al (1992) Interleukin-1 receptor antagonist circulates in the experimental inflammation and human disease. Blood 79:2196
86. Slotman GJ, Quinn JV, Wry PC et al (1997) Unopposed interleukin 1 is necessary for increased plasma cytokine and eicosanoid levels to develop in severe sepsis. Ann Surg 226:77
87. Kusuhara H, Matsuyuki H, Okumoto T (1997) Effects of nonsteroidal anti-inflammatory drugs on interleukin-1 receptor antogonist production in cultured peripheral blood mononuclear cells. Prostaglandins 54:795
88. De Bont ES, de Leij LH, Okken A et al (1995) Increased plasma concentrations of interleukin 1 receptor antagonist in neonatal sepsis. Pediatr Res 37:626
89. Endo S, Inada K, Yamada Y et al (1996) Plasma levels of interleukin 1 receptor antagonist and severity of illness in patients with burns. J Med 27:57
90. Shito M, Wakabayashi G, Ueda M et al (1997) Interleukin-1 receptor blockade reduces tumor necrosis factor production, tissue injury, and mortality after hepatic ischemia/reperfusion in the rat. Transplantation 63:143
91. Colagiovanni DB, Shopp GM (1996) Evaluation of interleukin-1 receptor antagonist and tumor necrosis factor binding protein in a rodent abscess model of host resistance. Immunopharmacol Immunotoxicol 18:397
92. Opal SM, Fisher CJ Jr, Dhainaut J-FA et al (1997) Confirmatory interleukin 1 receptor antagonist trial in severe sepsis: A phase III, randomized, double-blinded, placebo controlled, multicenter trial. Crit Care Med 25:1115

93. Mantovani A, Musio M, Ghezzi P et al (1998) Regulation of inhibitory pathways of the interleukin-1 system. Ann NY Acad Sci 840:338
94. De Waal Malefyt R, Abrams J, Bennet B et al (1991) Interleukin-10 inhibits cytokine synthesis by human monocytes: an autoregulatory role of IL-10 produced by monocytes. J Exp Med 174:1209
95. Marie C, Pitton C, Fitting C, Cavaillon JM (1996) IL-10 and IL-4 synergize with TNF alpha to induce IL-1ra production by human neutrophils. Cytokine 8:147
96. Marchant A, Deviere B, Byl B et al (1994) Interleukin 10 production during septicemia. Lancet 343:707
97. Derkx B, Marchant M, Goldman R et al (1995) High levels of interleukin 10 during the initial phase of fulminant meningococcal septic shock. J Infect Dis 171:229
98. Parsons PE, Moss M, Vannice JL et al (1997) Circulating Il-1ra and IL-10 levels are increased but do not predict the development of acute respiratory distress syndrome in at risk patients. Am J Respir Crit Care Med 155:1469
99. Marchant A, Bruyns C, Vandenabelle P et al (1994) IL-10 controls IFN-gamma and TNF production by activated macrophages. Eur J Immunol 24:1167
100. Rogy MA, Auffenberg T, Espat NJ et al (1995) Human tumor necrosis factor receptor and interleukin 10 gene transfer in the mouse reduces mortality to lethal endotoxemia and also attenuates local inflammatory responses. J Exp Med 181:2289
101. Marchant A, Vincent JL, Goldman M (1996) Interleukin 10 as a protective cytokine produced during sepsis. In: Morrison DC, Ryan JL (eds) Novel strategies in the treatment of sepsis, pp 301-311
102. Han J, Thompson FS, Beutler B (1990) Dexamethasone and pentoxifilline inhibit endotoxin induced cachectin tumor necrosis factor synthesis at separate points in the signaling pathway. J Exp Med 172:391
103. Zuckerman SH, Shellhaas J, Butler LD (1989) Differential regulation of lipopolysaccharide induced interleukin-1 and tumor necrosis factor and synthesis: effects of endogenous glucocorticoids and the role of the pituitary-adrenal axis. Eur J Immunol 19:301
104. Luedke CE, Cerami A (1990) Interferon gamma overcomes glucocorticoid suppression of cachectin/tumor necrosis factor biosynthesis by murine macrophages. J Clin Invest 86:1234
105. Ray A, LaForge KS, Sehgal PB (1990) On the mechanism for efficient repression of the interleukin-6 promoter by glucocorticoids: Enhancer, TATA box, and RNA start site occlusion. Mol Cell Biol 10:5736
106. Brown EA, Dare HA, Marsh CB, Wewers MD (1996) The combination of endotoxin and dexamethasone induces type II interleukin-1 receptor in monocytes: a comparison to interleukin-1 beta and interleukin-1 receptor antagonist. Cytokine 8:828
107. Horai R, Asano M, Sudo K et al (1988) Production of mice deficient in genes for IL-1 alpha, Il-1 beta, Il-1 alpha/beta, and Il-1 receptor antagonist shows that Il-1 beta is crucial in turpentine induced fever development and glucocorticoid secretion. J Exp Med 187:1463
108. Bernton EW, Beach JE, Holaday JW et al (1997) Release of multiple hormones by direct action of interleukin 1 on pituitary cells. Science 230:519
109. Berkenbosch F, van Oers J, del Rey A et al (1987) Corticotropin-releasing factor producing neurons in the rat activated by interleukin 1. Science 238:534
110. Lumpkin MD (1987) The regulation of ACTH secretion by IL-1. Science 238:452
111. Sapolsky R, Rivier C, Yamamot G et al (1987) Interleukin 1 stimulates the secretion of hypothalamic corticotropin-releasing factor. Science 238:522
112. Bernardini R, Kamilaris TC, Calogero AE et al (1990) Interactions between tumor necrosis factor alpha, hypothalamic corticotropin-releasing hormone, and adrenocorticotropin secretion in the rat. Endocrinology 126:2876
113. Gwosdow AR (1995) Mechanisms of interleukin 1 induced hormone secretion from rat adrenal gland. Endocr Res 21:25
114. Barber AE, Coyle SM, Marano MA et al (1993) Glucocorticoid therapy alters hormonal and cytokine response to endotoxin in man. J Immunol 150:1999

115. Joyce DA, Steer JH, Kloda A (1996) Dexamethasone antagonizes IL-4 and IL-10 induced release of IL-1 ra by monocytes but augments IL-4, Il-10, and TGF beta induced suppression of TNF alpha release. J Interferon Cytokine Res 16:511
116. Sauer J, Castren M, Hopfner U et al (1996) Inhibition of lipopolysaccharide induced monocyte interleukin-1 receptor antagonist synthesis by cortisol: involvement of mineralcorticoid receptor. J Clin Endocrinol Metab 81:73
117. Natanson C (1997) Anti-inflammatory therapies to treat sepsis and septic shock: A reassessment. Crit Care Med 25:1095
118. Pastores SM, Hasko G, Vizi ES, Kvetan V (1996) Cytokine production and its manipulation by vasoactive drugs. New Horiz 4:252
119. Van der Poll T, Jansen J, Endert E et al (1994) Noradrenaline inhibits lipopolysaccharide-induced tumor necrosis factor and interleukin 6 production in human whole blood. Infect Immun 62:2046
120. Van der Poll T, Braxton C, Coyle SM et al (1995) Effect of epinephrine on cytokine release during human endotoxemia. Surg Forum 46:102
121. Hamilton G, Hofbauer S, Hamilton B (1992) Endotoxin, TNF-α, interleukin 6 and parameters of the cellular immune system in patients with intraabdominal sepsis. Scand J Infect Dis 24:361

Injury, Inflammation, Sepsis - Is There a Natural, Organized and Sequential Progression of Neuroendocrine, Metabolic and Cytokine Mediator Events Leading to Organ System Failure?

A.E. BAUE

The title of my discussion contains a rhetorical question and the answer to a rhetorical question is always no. If the answer to the question was yes, the presenter, writer, author, or I would have said – "The natural organized – progression" indicates that I or he believed that there was such a thing.

The questions I will review are: 1) Is there a system to deal with injury? 2) Is it orderly and can we ever completely understand it? The answer to the first question is yes, there is a system, and it seems to be organized and appropriate but only for a moderate injury. It also seems to be orderly and connected after a moderate injury at least as we presently understand it. With severe or overwhelming injury there seems to be a biologic disintegration and the system is disorderly or out of control (Table 1). As to understanding it, we may never completely understand it if the system is out of control or if we apply conventional scientific homeostatic thinking. Let's review the evidence.

Table 1.

Extent of injury	Neuroendocrine, metabolic, cytokine and immune responses
Minimal surgery; laparoscopy, thoracoscopy, inguinal hernia repair; no large incision into a body cavity	Minimal and appropriate; little change in the homeostatic thermostatic
Major surgery and non-life threatening injury; a large incision in a body cavityor multisystem injury	Major changes but they seem to be interrelated and coordinated; homeostasis as we understand it seems evident
Life-threatening injuries, operations or illnesses	Biologic chaos - dyshomeostasis; the individual is overwhelmed by the multiplicity of changes which become self destructive

The first bit of evidence comes from how much injury a normal individual will tolerate without therapy. Sir Astley Cooper in 1838 described the enigma of injured soldiers dying without significant external blood loss, severe pain or gross injury [1]. Often the injury or insult seemed small in relationship to the profound effect (shock) on the patient. John Collins Warren provided a clinical description of this dilemma in 1895 [2]:

> A patient is brought into the hospital with a compound comminuted fracture or with a dis-location of the hip added to other injuries, where the bleeding has been slight. As the litter is gently deposited on the floor, he makes no effort to move or look about him. He lies staring at the surgeon with an expression of complete indifference as to this condition. There is no movement of muscles; and the eyes, which are deeply sunken in their pockets, have a weird, uncanny look. The features are pinched and the face shrunken. A cold, clam-my sweat exudes from the pores of the skin which has an appearance of profound anaemia. The lips are bloodless and the fingers and nails are blue. The pulse is almost im-perceptible; a weak thread-like stream may however be detected in the radial artery. The thermometer, placed in the rectum, registers 96° or 97° F. The muscles are not paralyzed anywhere, but the patient seems disinclined to make any muscular effort. Even respiratory movements seem for the time to be reduced to a minimum. Occasionally the patient may feebly throw about one of his limbs and give vent to a hoarse weak groan. There is no in-sensibility (coma is not observed in cases of shock), but he is strangely apathetic, and seems to realize but imperfectly the full meaning of the questions put to him. It is of no use to attempt an operation until appropriate remedies have brought about a reaction. The pulse, however, does not respond; it grows feebler and finally disappears. This "momen-tary pause in the act of death" is soon followed by a grim reality. A postmortem examina-tion reveals no visible changes in the internal organs.

Thus, a compound comminuted fracture of the femur with blood loss into the major large muscles of the thigh is sufficient to put a patient into shock and to produce death in an otherwise normal young person. Thus, the maximum amount of blood that an individual can lose without medical attention and thera-py is between 1,000 and 1,500 ml. When we give blood as a blood donor, this is usually only about 400 ml, so it will be the equivalent of donating three pints of blood and from this it will be unlikely that any of us would recover without treatment, particularly an intravenous infusion.

With modern therapy, patients are able to survive very serious illnesses or have major operations with a mortality that is very low. How do our biologic re-sponses to injury help with this?

The response and phases of injury

The metabolic and neuroendocrine responses to injury are important parts of the stress reaction. Teleologically, they improve the chances of survival from severe illness or injury. The objectives of this sequence are to maintain blood flow, oxygen delivery and organ perfusion and mobilize new substrates [3] for healing and recovery. Knowledge of these events and their clinical manifestations and observation of the patient's response help in patient care [3].

Injuries and major operations are similar in their pathophysiological threat. The term "injury" will be considered here to include the result of an event such as a motor vehicle accident or a planned elective, but still traumatic procedure in the operating room. The extent of injuries, the number of organs involved, the suddenness of the event, whether or not a body cavity has been entered or damaged, and the unplanned experience of trauma will differ in each patient but the biologic response is similar. The magnitude of the response varies according to the severity of the injury. A clean elective operation produces a level of stress beyond that associated with the fasting, resting state. Stress produced by multisystem injury, however, is much greater. The nervous, endocrine and immune systems interact to adapt to tissue injury, infection and inflammation with a dynamic, everchanging metabolic response. These changes were called the maladie post-operatoir by Leriche [4], the general alarm reaction by Selye [5], and the vegetativ Gesamtumschaltung by Hoff [6].

An acute phase response to inflammation, infection or physical trauma is characterized by fever, changes in vascular permeability, and changes in the biosynthetic and catabolic profiles of many organs.

There are four phases in the response to injury as originally described by Moore [7]. The first phase begins at the time of injury or, for an elective operation, during the preparation for the operation, when the patient stops oral intake, becomes anxious about the procedure and receives preoperative medication. The injury phase normally lasts two to five days, depending upon the magnitude of the injury and the presence or absence of complications. In normal convalescence in the second phase the turning point is a transient period marked physiologically by a "turning off" of the neuroendocrine response and clinically by the patient's appearing to get well. The third phase involves gain in muscular strength and in positive nitrogen balance. The fourth phase involves gain in weight and body fat and a positive caloric balance. Early expressions for these phases were the "ebb and flow" of Cuthbertson with "ebb" referring to the injury phase and "flow" referring to the recovery phase [8].

An excessive response leading to death has also been called "necrobiosis". These patterns are specific to trauma and do not occur in the same way in medical patients with sepsis.

The injury phase

The stimuli of injury

Several stimuli mediate the biologic response to injury, tending to reset the homeostatic thermostat at a higher metabolic and circulatory rate and a higher level of functioning. Pain, fear, fatigue, anaesthesia, drugs, immobilization and transient starvation produce only minor or short-term changes. Following an inguinal hernia repair with local anaesthesia, for example, the patient can be discharged from the hospital shortly thereafter with little change having occurred in the biologic thermostat. The systemic response to such a minor injury is minimal because the operation is on the surface of the body with local anaesthesia and none of the body cavities are entered. A similar response can also follow procedures performed within body cavities by thoracoscopic or laparoscopic approaches. The incisions required for such invasive procedures are so small that the response to injury is minimal and the patient can often be discharged within a day or two anticipating an uneventful convalescence. Tissue injury accompanied by necrosis, sepsis, shock and other aspects of ischaemia produce more striking effects. The afferent pathways with injury are shown in Fig. 1.

The efferent pathways from the cortex to the thalamus out to the periphery are shown in Fig. 2. The wound must be considered an organ – the area of injury, incision and operated organs – hence it functions somewhat independently as it calls on the rest of the body for support. The wound establishes a high biologic priority for itself and initiates many changes in the metabolic response to injury providing afferent stimuli to the central nervous system, efferent stimuli to the liver, temperature control center and elsewhere. The mediators come from cells in the wound such as macrophages, monocytes, neutrophils, endothelial cells and others. These mediators have autocrine and paracrine activity. Plus, the wound itself initiates the inflammatory response; infection, if it occurs, exaggerates that response [9].

In addition to the hypothalamic, pituitary, adrenal responses with increased ADH, CRH, ACTH, and catecholamines, there are also increases in angiotensin 2, aldosterone, the endorphins and various neurotransmitters. Glucagon is increased and insulin is depressed so that it does not respond to appropriate levels of hyperglycaemia.

Physiologic correlates

The physiologic correlates of the neuroendocrine response during the injury phase include: 1) blood pressure and cardiac output maintenance by cardiovascular compensation and capillary refilling; 2) salt and water retention to maintain vascular and extracellular fluid volume; 3) increased metabolic rate (hypermetabolism); 4) altered metabolism with insulin resistance, hyperglycaemia, gluconeogenesis, excess catabolism, and negative nitrogen balance, with release of intracellular components; 5) mobilization of fat; 6) beginning of wound healing; and 7) immunomodulation [3].

Clinical correlates

The clinical correlates of this injury phase are that the patient is quiet, lethargic, appears ill and is not interested in his or her surroundings or appearance. This is a result of pain, and β-endorphin, enkephalin and IL-1 production. The pulse in-

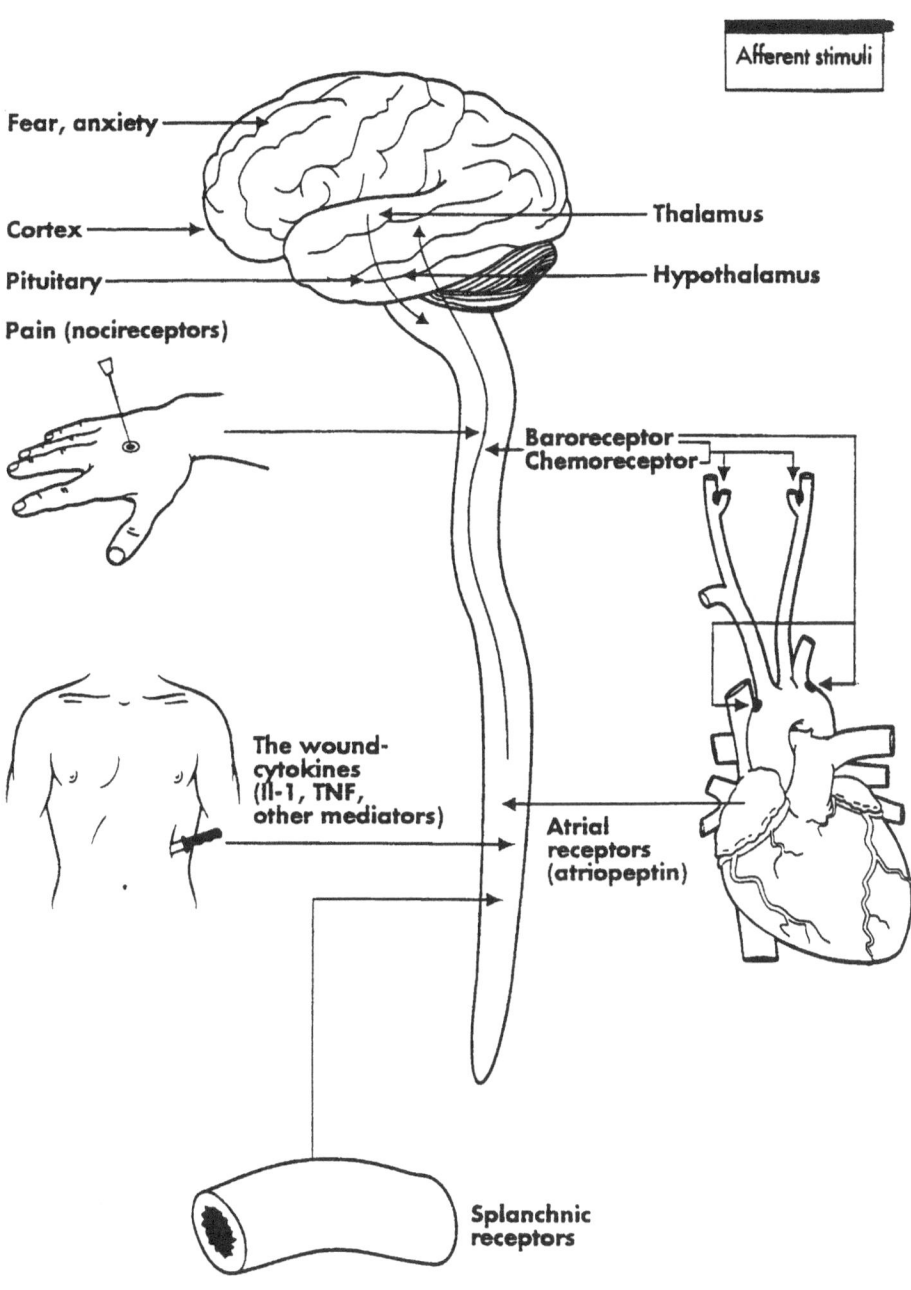

Fig. 1.

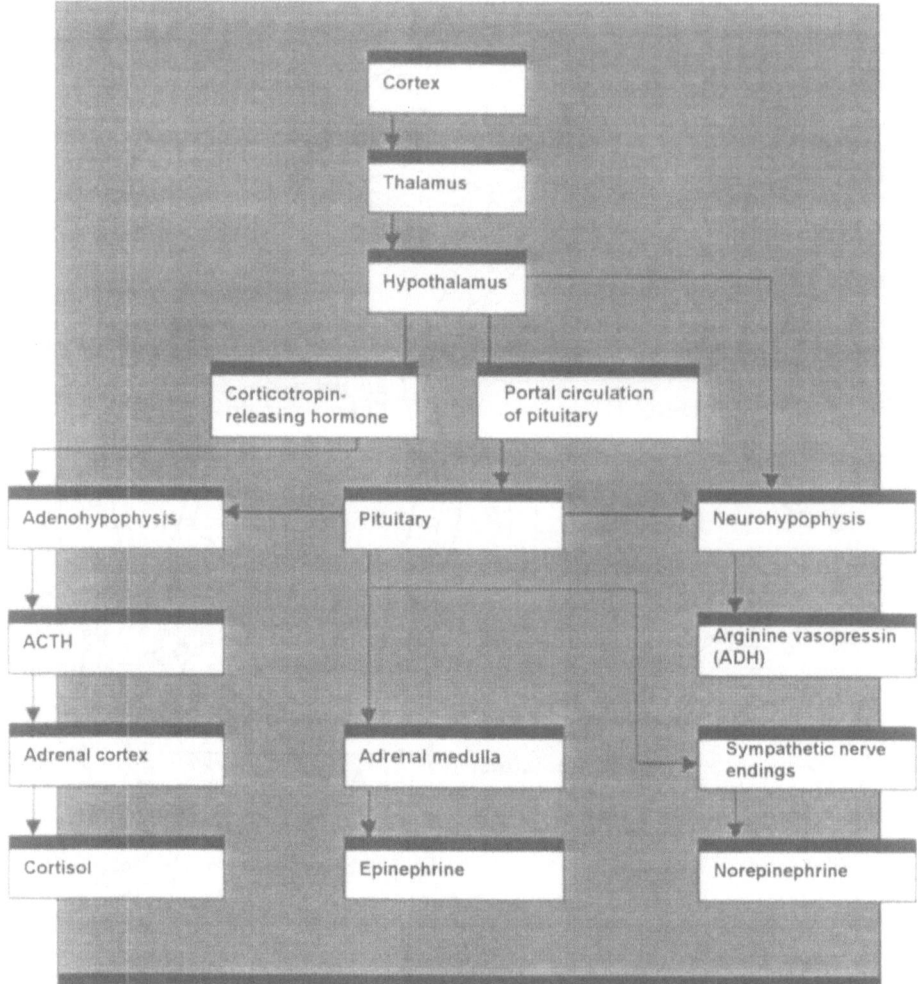

Fig. 2.

creases modestly, body temperature increases with a low-grade fever, oliguria develops, appetite decreases, the gastrointestinal tract and peristalsis are quiet and pain is present [3].

The turning point and later phases

If the patient becomes stable, homeostasis is adequate, the wound is controlled and no complications occur, then the turning point is reached in which the entire neuroendocrine metabolic response is turned off. The patient begins to look better and begins further convalescence. This leads then to the anabolic phase which begins immediately after the turning point, particularly when the patient can take nourishment, and goes on for some weeks replacing loss of lean body mass or muscle. Late anabolism, the fourth phase, occurs some time later and entails positive caloric and carbon balance. Fat stores are replaced and the patient returns to a total normal state. Depending upon the magnitude of the operation or injury, this may take from three to six months [3].

Therapeutic principles

Prompt operative management is the key to recovery. Correcting blood loss, repairing injured organs, supporting damaged organs, and closing wounds should stop the wounding stimulus and shorten the injury phase.

Careful surgical technique will minimize tissue necrosis and decrease the chances of infection in the wound and elsewhere. Debridement, irrigation, cleaning, and stopping continued pleural, peritoneal, bone, or muscle contamination are critical. Minimal surgical procedures decrease the response to injury [10, 11].

Epidural or spinal anaesthesia and agents such as fentanyl and morphine may decrease the response to injury by decreasing the cortisol, cAMP, and glucose responses [12, 13]. Epidural analgesia also prevents the sensitization of the spinal cord by pain. The effect may be enough to decrease morbidity. In one study, a combination of prednisolone, epidural analgesia and indomethacin decreased the stress response in patients having colon operations [14]. The combined use of thoracic epidural analgesia and blockade of glucagon (and insulin) by somatostatin and blockade of cortisol by etomidate prevented the hepatic catabolic effects after cholecystectomy [15]. This helps define the mechanisms of injury more than it directs therapy. The physiologic response to stress can be attenuated by deep anaesthesia with sufentanil and postoperative analgesia with sufentanil and postoperative analgesia with high doses of opioids in high-risk neonates having cardiac surgery.

Pain relief, intravenous fluids to compensate for third space requirements, and mobilization are important. Nutritional support decreases total protein loss. Early postinjury enteral feeding should be provided whenever possible, particularly if the patient will not be able to resume oral intake within three to four days or is severely hypermetabolic [16]. Additives such as glutamine, arginine, omega-3 fatty acids, branched-chain amino acids, and antioxidants (vitamins C, A, and E and glutathione) may decrease infection and enhance immune function [17].

Total parenteral or enteral nutrition, however, cannot abolish the hypermetabolic, hyperglycaemic response to catabolic hormones. Hormonal manipulations are being evaluated with anabolic hormones such as exogenous insulin, growth hormone, and insulin-like growth hormone which may reduce protein loss, preserve body composition, increase strength, and decrease infection [18]. The value of these agents is still being investigated so they are not yet recommended for general clinical use in such patients.

In patients with extreme hypermetabolism (e.g., burns) the cardiovascular effects can be blunted by β-adrenergic blockade. Metoprolol, a β-2 blocking agent, has been used to decrease the hyperdynamic response in burned children [19].

Aberrancies

Some years ago we studied altered hormonal activity in severely ill patients after injury or sepsis. All such patients in the intensive care unit initially had low normal levels of T4 and of low T3 with normal thyroid stimulating hormone (TSH) levels. This has been called the low T3 syndrome and is quite consistent with just being sick. In surviving patients these levels increased to normal before leaving the intensive care unit. The patients who died showed no further decreases before death [20].

Corticotropin, cortisol, prolactin and growth hormone levels were normal throughout the study in all patients. Catecholamine levels were high initially and decreased in surviving patients. Epinephrine levels increased greatly in non-survivors before death and the norephinephrine-epinephrine ratio decreased from 5:7:1 to 2:1. After protirelin (thyroid-releasing hormone) stimulation, the TSH level increased either minimally or not at all in six patients who eventually died. This indicates hypothalamic, pituitary dysregulation or suppression and altered release and/or peripheral metabolism of T4. Whether this represents a deficiency of thyroid hormone for cell and organ function has not been established.

There are many associations and interactions between the neuroendocrine and immune systems. These have been reviewed thoroughly by Wygent and Blalock [21].

Self destruction

The massive neuroendocrine, metabolic and mediator response that occurs with major trauma shows that the supposedly "protective" biologic responses to injury can be self-destructive [22]. The pro-inflammatory mediators IL-1, TNF, Il-6, IL-8 and IL-12 all play a role. The anti-inflammatory mediators attempt to control the situation and include IL-1ra, IL-4, IL-10, IL-11, IL-13, transforming growth factor β, bactericidal permeability increasing protein and other factors.

The response to injury is teleologically designed to allow the individual to recover without treatment. If the injury is more severe, then the response is overwhelming and difficult to control. This has been called a "horror autotoxicus" [23], a term originated by Paul Ehrlich many years ago to suggest a self-destructive or autoimmune process [24].

We would like to think that this response is a highly organized, integrated and controlled biologic process. Lewis Thomas, however, provides evidence that these responses get out of control and cause harm to the individual [25]. He states: "I suspect that the host was caught up in mistaken, inappropriate and unquestionably self-destructive mechanism by the very multiplicity of defenses available to him which do not seem to have been designed to operate in net coordination with each other. The end result is not defense, it is an agitated committee-directed harum-scarum effort to make war".

Variations in patients

We are now being told about differences in patients which may have a great influence on the results of therapy. Genetic differences in the cytokine response to sepsis have been described and discussed [26, 27]. Marked preoperative differences in immunity to endotoxin (as measured by endotoxin core antibody - Endocab) were found in cardiac surgical patients [28]. Low levels predicted adverse postoperative outcomes. This IgM Endocab study indicates that prior immune history is important in response to stress. Prior exposure indicates the ability to respond to various antigens. This may not only be for endotoxin or gram negative infections but for other exposures as well. Could it be that these individuals have a healthier and better trained immune response?

In all standard, randomized, prospective, double-blinded trials there is usually a statement such as "There were no differences in characteristics of the patients in age, sex, cause and severity of sepsis or of injury in the control and the treated groups". Now the question must be asked: How do they know that the groups are comparable? Their previous health status may be known, the injury or severity score may be known, but how do we know what exposure they have had and what their immune response may be?

Rook and Stanford remind us that exposure to antigens is important in maintaining immunologic health [29]. Modern life has decreased that exposure. They suggest the possibility of two "input deprivation states". The first of these (the imbalance state) involves inadequate primary Th (Th_1) activity leading to an incorrect cytokine balance. This could derive from vaccination by a Th_2-mediated antibody dependent mechanism which denies the immune system the learning experience of infections through a Th_1-mediated pathway.

The second deprivation involves a failure to fine tune the T-cell repertoire in relationship to epitopes that are cross-reactive between cells and microorganisms (the Uneducated T-cell Regulation State).

Summary

The biologic response to injury serves to maintain the viability of the organism under adverse circumstances. An understanding of this response, its variations and its pathologic distortions allow a physician to treat the injured patient properly. The organism copes with modest injury by maintaining perfusion of vital organs, mobilizing body water and altering metabolism to heal the injury, a response essential for survival. An inflammatory response is necessary. When the injury is overwhelming, however, the response also becomes overwhelming and potentially destructive. The consequences may include the following:

1. The altered immune response may increase susceptibility to infection at a time when the patient most needs protection from infection;

2. Excessive catabolism and proteolysis can jeopardize a patient's survival;

3. Activation of normally protective mechanisms or enzyme cascades, when present in excessive amounts, such as white blood cells, complement and other factors may damage remote organs;

4. Tissue necrosis and its breakdown products may depress the function of organs such as the myocardium;

5. Salt and water retention that cannot be controlled produce generalized oedema;

6. The prolonged effects of shock and ischaemia may increase organ susceptibility to damage from an ischaemia-reperfusion injury;

7. The effects of infection may be devastating and the final potentially lethal insult.

The impact of the new integrative or nonlinear biology will also change some of these concepts.

References

1. Cooper A (1838) A dictionary of practical surgery, 7th edn. Longmans, London
2. Warren JC (1895) Surgical pathology and therapeutics. WB Saunders, Philadelphia
3. Baue AE (1990) Metabolic and neuroendocrine response to injury. In: Baue AE (ed) Multiple organ failure: Patient care and prevention. Mosby Year Book, St. Louis
4. Leriche R, cited by Lambret O, Driessens J (1937) Les modifications humorales post-operatoires: Pathogenie-traitement: Recherches personelles. J Int Chir 2:223-265
5. Selye H (1946) The general adaptation syndrome and the alarm reaction. J Clin Endocrinol Metabol 6:117-230
6. Hoff F (1930) Unspezifische Therapie und natürliche Abwehrvorgange. Springer, Berlin
7. Moore FD (1959) Metabolic care of the surgical patient. WB Saunders, Philadelphia
8. Cuthbertson DP (1942) Post-shock metabolic response. Lancet 242:433-437
9. Baue AE (1990) The wound as an organ. In: Baue AE (ed) Multiple organ failure: Patient care and prevention. Mosby Year Book, St. Louis
10. Kloosterman T, von Blomberg M, Borgstein P (1994) Unimpaired immune functions after laparoscopic cholecystectomy. Surgery 115:424

11. Ueo H, Honda H, Adachi M (1994) Minimal increase in serum interleukin-6 levels during laparoscopic cholecystectomy. Am J Surg 168:358
12. Smeets HJ, Kievitz J, Dulfer FT (1993) Endocrine-metabolic response to abdominal aortic surgery: a randomized trial of general anesthesia versus general plus epidural anesthesia. World J Surg 17:601-607
13. Glerup H, Heindorff H, Flyvbjerg H (1995) Elective laparoscopic cholecystectomy nearly abolishes the postoperative hepatic catabolic stress response. Ann Surg 221:214-219
14. Schulze S, Sommer P, Bigler D (1992) Effect of combined prednisolone, epidural analgesia, and indomethacin on the systemic response after colonic surgery. Arch Surg 127:325
15. Heindorff H, Schulze S, Mogensen T (1992) Hormonal and neural blockade prevents the postoperative increase in amino acid clearance and urea synthesis. Surgery 111:543
16. Moore FA, Moore E, Kudsk K (1994) Clinical benefits of an immune-enhancing diet for early postinjury enteral feeding. J Trauma 37:607
17. Demling RH, Lalonde C, Ikegami K (1994) Physiologic support of the septic patient. Surg Clin North Am 74:637
18. Byrne TA, Morrissey T, Gatzon C (1993) Anabolic therapy with growth hormone accelerates protein gain in surgical patients requiring nutritional rehabilitation. Ann Surg 218:400
19. Herndon DN, Nguyen T, Wolfe R (1994) Lipolysis in burned patients is stimulated by the β-2 receptor for catecholamines. Arch Surg 129:1301
20. Baue AE, Gunther B, Hartl W et al (1984) Altered hormonal activity in severely ill patients after injury or sepsis. Arch Surg 119:1125-1132
21. Wygent DA, Blalock JE (1995) Associations between the neuroendocrine and immune systems. J Leukoc Biol 57:137-150
22. Baue AE (1993) Host defense system failure. In: Baue AE (ed) Multiple organ failure: Patient care and prevention. Mosby Year Book, St. Louis
23. Baue AE (1990) Multiple organ failure: Patient care and prevention. Mosby Year Book, St. Louis
24. Ehrlich P, Morgenroth J (1901) II: Ueber-Hämolysins. Fünfte Mitheilung. Berl Klin Wochenschr 38:251-257
25. Thomas L (1970) Adaptive aspects of inflammation. Presented at third symposium of the International Inflammation Club. Published by Upjohn Co, Kalamazoo
26. Stüber F, Petersen M, Bokelmann F, Schade U (1996) A genomic polymorphism within the tumor necrosis factor locus influences plasma tumor necrosis factor-α concentrations and outcome of patients with severe sepsis. Crit Care Med 24(3):381-387
27. Zehnbauer BA, Buchman TG (1996) Clinical molecular genetics and critical care medicine. Crit Care Med 24(3):373-375
28. Bennett-Guerrero E, Ayuso L, Hamilton-Davies C et al (1997) Relationship of preoperative anti-endotoxin core antibodies and adverse outcomes following cardiac surgery. JAMA 277 (8):646-650
29. Rook GAW, Stanford JL (1998) Give us this day our daily germs. Immunol Today 19: 113-116

Genetic Predisposition to Sepsis and Organ Failure

B.A. ZEHNBAUER, B.D. FREEMAN, T.G. BUCHMAN

Sepsis and organ failure continue to challenge practitioners of critical care and their patients. The purpose of this brief review is to explore emerging information about genetic predisposition to sepsis and organ failure. For this discussion, we will define a continuum from sepsis through organ failure to represent a set of responses to infection and ischemia which, left unchecked, ordinarily results in severe disability or death. These responses are presently thought to represent a dysregulated synthesis of pro- and anti-inflammatory responses chronicled elsewhere in this volume.

Genes, genotypes and phenotypic responses

In this era of molecular biology, it is deceptively easy to describe a gene in terms of its DNA sequence. It is well to recall that, until the Beadle-Tatum experiments which advanced the "one gene-one enzyme" hypothesis, substantial controversy raged regarding the structure-function interrelationships among genes, phenotypes, nucleic acids and proteins [3]. Whereas a particular piece of DNA contains the nucleotide sequences coding for particular gene products (the "structural" portions of the gene), that particular piece of DNA also contains untranslated sequence which may ("cis-acting elements") or may not (introns, "junk DNA") regulate the expression of the structural gene's product. Moreover, relatively distant segments of DNA ("enhancers") may directly affect expression of the structural gene's product as is the case, for example, for the β-globin gene. Structurally normal genes may contain common and normal variants ("alleles") which give rise to unusual phenotypes when their expression depends significantly on the state of regulators of gene expression such as trans-acting "factors" or allosteric modifiers. The key question we seek to answer in this brief chapter is, "are there genetic variants which can regulate severity and even predict outcome in sepsis and inflammation?". To address this question, we need to concern ourselves not only with the genes coding for the pro and anti-inflammatory proteins but also with known and even unknown regulators of the expression and activity of those proteins. Importantly, rather than biological mechanism, we will focus exclusively on correlation with genetic variance. In this context, it is appropriate to concern ourselves primarily with genetic markers, recognizing that markers may be located in DNA sequences within, adjacent to, or quite distant from inflammatory genes.

We define a DNA polymorphism as two or more alternative genotypes in a population, each at a frequency greater than that which could be attributed to mutation [4]. Usually polymorphic alleles are present in a population at a frequency of at least 1%. These markers exhibit mendelian inheritance patterns and are widely distributed throughout the genome. For the last 20 years DNA polymorphisms have become increasingly important in the construction of human genetic maps and are relatively easy to localize on the physical map of the human genome.

There are several "easy-to-localize" types of polymorphisms. RFLP's are site polymorphisms which result from variations in DNA sequence that create or destroy specific cleavage sites for restriction endonucleases. This variability is detected as a change in the size of DNA fragments produced by cutting with restriction enzymes. This site alteration results in two different versions or alleles for the marker region. Three different patterns are possible for a site polymorphism: two copies with the site (+/+), two copies without the site (–/–), or heterozygous (+/– or –/+) for one copy of each allele. VNTR's and microsatellites are length polymorphisms that differ by varying the number of repeated copies of a consensus DNA sequence between two consistent restriction enzyme sites. As the number of repeated copies varies, a large number of differently sized polymorphic alleles result and generate genetic heterozygosity with high frequency. The diversity or informativeness of a polymorphism is based in its ability to distinguish the DNA from individuals in the population as different thus the potential to generate many different patterns is key to the marker's utility. Polymerase chain reaction techniques using primer sequences which flank the polymorphism make mapping and diagnostic screening with microsatellite markers relatively quick and straightforward.

Most gene/disease correlations have been made between the clinical symptoms of the disease (phenotype) and the polymorphic marker pattern or length (genotype) by linkage analysis in family studies. Since "families" typically do not sustain sepsis or organ failure, it is necessary to build the relationships based on statistical association in population studies. These genetic association studies do not examine familial inheritance patterns but rather are case-control studies comparing unrelated affected and unaffected individuals from a population. Positive association is defined as a concurrence between disease and marker alleles within a population that is greater than predicted by chance [1, 2]. Association studies using polymorphic DNA markers are understandably most significant when the genetic variations have functional significance and are related to the biology of the disorder, and therefore most students of sepsis have initially focused on the genes of the inflammatory response.

Before discussing the data, it is important to remember two features of association studies. First, marker/disease gene associations are usually not equivalent to *physical* linkage. Second, the strength of the marker/gene association technique lies in the composition of the healthy control population which must precisely represent the same composition as the population from which the patients are drawn. The healthy group must be entirely typical of the patient population in order to avoid the "founder effect" artifacts which have their roots in different allele frequencies inherent in different ethnic subgroups [1]. A study of the genotypes of the affected individuals and their parents provides an artificial internal control that is well matched for ethnic ancestry, a strategy that is frequently possible in younger (e.g. post-trauma) sepsis patients. Thus, genetic association within a population is a method for ascertaining genetic influences on disease phenotype when family studies are neither available nor feasible such as identification of genetic factors in the predisposition to inflammation or sepsis. As we shall see, DNA polymorphisms in several genes for inflammation functions produce stable variations in cytokine production which are positively associated with susceptibility to sepsis and multiple organ system failure.

Tumor necrosis factor

Genetic variation within the tumor necrosis factor (TNF) locus, one of the best-studied, polymorphic genes in inflammatory responses, has been important in determining susceptibility to, or severity of, a significant number of critical illnesses including infectious diseases and septic shock [5, 11]. The TNF α and TNF β gene cluster contains two polymorphic sites for the restriction enzyme Nco 1 (RFLP's): one located in the promoter region for TNF α and another in the first intron of TNF β [6]. A single base change (G $\rightarrow$ A at base pair -308 in TNF α and A $\rightarrow$ G at bp 1069 within the first intron of TNF β) creates or destroys the polymorphic scission site for this enzyme. The polymorphisms define 2 alternative alleles at each of these positions (TNF α A1 and A2 plus TNF β B1 and B2). Each allele with loss of an Nco 1 site (TNFA2 and TNFB2) correlates with increased synthesis of TNF and exacerbation of inflammatory responses [6]. Again, this does not imply that the polymorphism itself causes increased TNF expression but merely that it may be used as a marker to trace the occurrence of the allele and its possible correlation with specific clinical manifestations [1].

McGuire and colleagues [8] hypothesized that while cerebral malaria occurred in a small fraction of malaria patients, a critical determinant was thought to be an elevated level of TNF α associated with disease severity. Previous studies had shown a ten-fold higher plasma TNF α concentration in children with cerebral malaria compared to those with mild malaria. These workers molecularly characterized the presence and frequency of the TNFA2 allele in severely affected malaria patients and compared it to the allele frequency in both normal and mild malaria control patient populations. The frequency of A1/A2 heterozygotes was similar (0.16) in each of these groups. However, the frequency of TNFA2 homozygotes was several-fold higher in the subgroups of malaria patients exhibiting severe clinical symptoms. The data was consistent with an increased relative risk of 4 for cerebral malaria and 7 for death or severe neurological damage in TNFA2 homozygous individuals. This regulatory polymorphism of the TNF α gene affected the outcome of a severe infection.

Increased levels of TNF α also correlated with the severity of meningococcal disease (MD). Nadel and coworkers [9] investigated the distribution of the TNF α A1 and A2 alleles in children with fulminant MD. About 10-15% of patients with MD have meningococcal septicaemia with mortality rates of 20-60%. In this study TNFA1/A2 heterozygotes had an associated 2.5-fold increased risk of death from MD relative to children who did not possess the TNFA2 allele. The frequency of the TNFA2 allele in all populations was the same because TNFA2 did not alter the risk of acquiring the infection. Individuals with the TNFA2 allele had a genetic predisposition to secrete higher levels of TNF α. The presence of the TNFA2 allele increased their risk for a more severe clinical course.

Increased levels of tumor necrosis factor are also observed with the TNFB2 polymorphic allele. The presence of this marker correlated with an increased risk for multiple organ failure in ICU patients with severe sepsis as described by Stuber [7, 10]. The allele frequency of TNFB2 in all ICU patients was the same as in the normal control population but was positively associated with non-survival in ICU patients with severe sepsis (relative risk of 2.1). Thus the TNFB2 genotype predisposed these critically ill patients to a high risk of severe systemic inflammation and a poor outcome.

Interleukin-1 and its receptor antagonist

Stuber and colleagues also determined the possible association of polymorphic alleles of two other inflammation genes, interleukin 1 (IL-1 β) and interleukin 1 receptor antagonist (IL-1ra), in these same patients [10]. They concluded that the IL-1B A2 allele, which correlates with high IL-1 β secretion, was not a poor prognostic indicator because IL-1B A2 did not differ in incidence between patients in the ICU and normal controls *or* between survivors and non-survivors. A relatively uncommon polymorphic allele, IL-1ra A2, related to high production of the IL-1ra protein, also showed significantly higher frequency in patients with severe sepsis compared to normal controls. Patients who were homozygous for both TNFB2 and IL-1ra A2 were exclusively non-survivors. The findings suggest that all polymorphic genetic variants which confer increased inflammation gene expression do not confer poor prognosis. IL-1ra A2 may contribute to susceptibility to sepsis while TNFB2 predicts high risk for poor outcome in severe sepsis.

Other approaches

From this brief discussion of existing human studies, it is apparent that screening for polymorphisms is a "needle-in-a-haystack" approach to the search for human sepsis susceptibility genes. While future technological progress may eventually make it possible to "allelotype" large regions of each individual human's genome, such advances will not occur in the foreseeable future. For this reason, alternative approaches are required. One attractive approach is being pursued by DeMaio and colleagues [12] who have recognized that mouse models of sepsis are fairly accurate mimics of the human condition. They have taken advantage of extensive knowledge about mouse genetics and of a series of mouse strains ("recombinant inbred strains") which are genetically pure and distinct from one another. They have observed that these strains vary widely with respect to their mortality following a standardized septic insult. In principle, it should be possible to map sepsis susceptibility in mice using standard genetic techniques and then determine if the human homologues of the relevant mouse genetic loci do, in fact, regulate the outcome in human sepsis. Put differently, the mouse data will tell us in which regions of the haystack we are likely to find a needle or two.

References

1. Lander ES, Schork NJ (1994) Genetic dissection of complex traits. Science 265:2037-2048
2. Sparkes RS (1992) Human gene mapping, linkage, and association. In: King RA, Rotter JI, Motulsky AG (eds) The genetic basis of common diseases. Oxford University, New York
3. Hodge SE (1994) What association studies can and cannot tell us about the genetics of complex disease. Am J Med Gen 54:318-323
4. Thompson MW, McInnes RR, Willard HF (1991) Genetics in medicine, 5th edn. WB Saunders, Philadelphia
5. Kunkel SL, Lukacs N, Streiter RM (1996) Cytokines and inflammatory disease. In: Sirica AE (ed) Cellular and molecular pathogenesis. Lippincott, Philadelphia, pp 23-35
6. Wilson AG, di Giovine FS, Duff GW (1995) Genetics of tumor necrosis factor-alpha in autoimmune, infectious, and neoplastic diseases. J Inflamm 45:1-12
7. Stuber F, Petersen M, Bokelmann F, Schade U (1996) A genomic polymorphism within the tumor necrosis factor locus influences plasma tumor necrosis factor-alpha concentrations and outcome in patients with severe sepsis. Crit Care Med 24:381-384
8. McGuire W, Hill AVS, Allsopp CEM et al (1994) Variation in the TNF-promoter region associated with susceptibility to cerebral malaria. Nature 371:508-511
9. Nadel S, Newport MJ, Booy R, Levin M (1996) Variation in the tumor necrosis factor a gene promoter region may be associated with death from meningococcal disease. J Infect Dis 174: 878-880
10. Stuber F, Fang X-M, Putensen C, Hoeft A (1998) Genomic polymorphisms of interleukin-1 RA and tumor necrosis factor define an extended haplotype for risk assessment in severe sepsis. Crit Care Med 26[Suppl]:A29
11. Seitzer U, Swider C, Stuber F et al (1997) Tumor necrosis factor alpha promoter gene polymorphism in sarcoidosis. Cytokine 9:787-790
12. DeMaio A, Mooney ML, Matesic L et al (1998) Genetic contribution to the inflammatory response. Shock 9[Suppl 1]:27 (abstract)

Regulation of the Lung Inflammatory Response

P.A. WARD, A.B. LENTSCH

Lung inflammatory responses in rat lung induced by deposition of IgG immune complexes are associated with complement activation, influx of neutrophils, activation of pulmonary macrophages and ensuing injury of the lung parenchyma [1]. Injury in this model is associated with extravascular leak of albumin, development of haemorrhage and damage of cellular and matrix constituents. Tissue injury is likely due to the combined effects of oxidants and proteases released from activated lung macrophages and from recruited neutrophils following a complex sequence of cellular and mediator interactions [2]. Essential to an understanding of these inflammatory events is the relationship between lung macrophage production of cytokines [such as tumor necrosis factor-alpha (TNFα) and interleukin-1 (IL-1)] and the response of the lung vasculature, the result of which is upregulation of endothelial adhesion molecules, including intercellular adhesion molecule-1 (ICAM-1) and E-selectin. We have found that these lung inflammatory reactions are carefully self-regulated. That is to say, the intensity of the inflammatory response builds up to a crescendo, peaking between 3-4 hours, then rapidly diminishes, as reflected by a reduction in vascular permeability, a cessation in haemorrhage and no further accumulation of neutrophils [3]. In some manner, then, these inflammatory responses are under regulatory control that ensures the potentially destructive inflammatory response will be contained.

Critical role of early response cytokines

To better understand how the lung inflammatory response is regulated, it is important to emphasize the role of the "early response" cytokines, which consist predominantly of TNFα and IL-1. These pro-inflammatory cytokines are products of lung macrophages which have been stimulated by intrapulmonary deposition of IgG immune complexes. These immune complexes also bring about the generation of complement activation products, including the anaphylatoxin, C5a, and the membrane attack complex (C5b-9) [4]. The combination of immune complexes interacting with lung macrophage Fc receptors (FcR) as well as immune complex Fc-induced activation of the complement system results in gene activation and enhanced generation of TNFα and IL-1 [5, 6]. These cytokines have the crucial role of stimulating lung vascular endothelial cells, bringing about gene activation and appearance of mRNA for ICAM-1 and E-selectin, followed by protein expression [5]. The appearance of E-selectin on lung vascular endothelial cells allows for engagement of E-selectin with its "counter receptors" (oligosaccharides with the sialyl Lewis^x motif) on surfaces of neutrophils, leading to E-selectin dependent "rolling" (intermittent adhesion) of neutrophils along the endothelial surfaces. The counter-receptors for these oligosaccharides are known to be P-selectin glycoprotein ligand-1 (PSGL-1) and E-selectin ligand-1 (ESL-1). Firm attachment of neutrophils to the vascular endothelium then occurs via engagement of endothelial ICAM-1 with the $β_2$ integrins, LFA-1 (CD11a/CD18) and Mac-1 (CD11b/CD18) on neutrophils. Subsequently, transmigration occurs via the influence of locally generated chemotactic factors including chemokines (IL-8 family of peptides) and C5a.

Complement activation products directly and indirectly influence expression of lung vascular adhesion molecules. For instance, C5a enhances lung macrophage production of TNFα in lung [7], while C5b-9 can interact with small amounts of TNFα to bring about synergistic expression of endothelial ICAM-1 and E-selectin [8]. C5a and C5b-9 can each directly cause upregulation of endothelial P-selectin [9-11]. The crucial linkage between TNFα and IL-1 with vascular adhesion molecule expression has been shown by the finding that, if either TNFα or IL-1 is blocked, there is greatly reduced expression of vascular ICAM-1, leading to diminished recruitment of neutrophils and reduced lung injury [5, 12]. As will be described below, one of the important functions of TNFα in lung is to bring about activation of nuclear factor kappa B (NFκB), a key transcriptional promoting factor which is required for initiation and propagation of maximal TNFα production and ICAM-1 expression on endothelial cells.

Activation by NFκB

It has been known for some time that most cell types contain NFκB, which may exist in a number of different dimeric combinations of proteins of the Rel family [13]. The most common and functionally significant form of NFκB is comprised of a heterodimeric complex of p50 and p65 subunits. This complex is retained in the cytosol of cells through interactions with members of the IκB protein family. In this configuration, IκB proteins bound to the NFκB complex mask the nuclear localization sequence of NFκB, thus preventing translocation of NFκB to the nuclear compartment and binding to DNA. Ordinarily in the course of cell activation a common member of the IκB family, IκBα, undergoes phosphorylation and ubiquination, which sets the stage for its proteolysis through the action of the 26S proteasome [14]. Upon disassociation from IκB, the NFκB complex can then gain entry into the nucleus where it binds to promoter sequences of DNA, resulting in transcriptional activation of relevant genes (e.g. TNFα and IL-1) [14]. Gene activation leading to expression of TNFα, IL-1 and endothelial adhesion molecules are just a few examples of products whose generation is NFκB-dependent. NFκB activation appears to be associated with the action of an intracellularly generated oxidant, in as much as a series of small molecular weight anti-oxidants have the ability to interfere with NFκB activation. Extracellular oxidants (such as H_2O_2) which readily gain access to the cytosol of cells will also induce activation of NFκB [15, 16]. Interventions that interfere with the process of NFκB translocation will thus reduce NFκB-dependent responses, causing reduced generation of TNFα and IL-1. As will be described below, it would appear that a key function of regulatory interleukins (IL's), which suppress inflammatory responses, is to inhibit the activation of NFκB.

Exogenous regulatory interleukins

Some time ago we discovered in the IgG immune complex model of lung injury that there was a group of IL's which, if exogenously applied by co-instillation with antibody to bovine serum albumin (anti-BSA) into lung, would cause substantial suppression of the lung inflammatory response. Using murine recombinant peptides, the first such IL's that were found to have these suppressive effects were IL-4 and IL-10 [17]. Under the experimental conditions employed, both IL-4 and IL-10 profoundly inhibited the lung inflammatory response by interfering with neutrophil recruitment. These outcomes required very low concentrations (ng quantities) of either IL-4 or IL-10. The next critical observation was that these IL's greatly suppressed lung production of TNFα. As predicted, there was substantially reduced upregulation of lung vascular ICAM-1, as demonstrated quantitatively by the use of ^{125}I-anti-rat-ICAM-1. For this type of analysis, binding of ^{125}I-anti-ICAM-1 to the lung vasculature was measured and compared to the binding of an irrelevant subclass-matched mouse IgG [17]. A comprehensive analysis of regulatory IL's in the lung inflammatory model revealed the following rank order for anti-inflammatory activity (from the most effective to the least potent): IL-10 = IL-13 > IL-4 >> IL-6 >> IL-12 [18]. One common theme for the effects of these IL's was the fact that they suppressed lung inflammation by reducing intrapulmonary production of TNFα. This, in turn, was associated with a substantial or complete reduction in the upregulation of lung vascular ICAM-1 and neutrophil recruitment. In the case of the lung model employed, it was determined that, except for IL-4, all of these regulatory IL's are expressed during the lung inflammatory response, as assessed by appearance of mRNA and protein in lung extracts.

Regulatory roles of endogenous IL-6 and IL-10

In the IgG immune complex model, we have cloned rat IL-6 and IL-10 and have developed reagents to detect mRNA's and related proteins. Polyclonal antibody to IL-6 or IL-10 has been used for *in vivo* blockade [19, 20]. From these experiments, the role of endogenously produced IL-6 and IL-10 in regulating the intensity of the lung inflammatory response has been assessed. As indicated above, for what ever reason, IL-4 is not expressed in lung under the experimental conditions employed. Neither IL-4 mRNA nor protein could be detected in lung extracts. Blocking antibody to rat IL-4 did not have any protective effects in the lung inflammatory response, even though this antibody was found to be protective in collagen-induced arthritis in rats [21]. It was therefore concluded that IL-4 is not an endogenous regulator of lung inflammation under the conditions employed. However, the findings were quite different for IL-10 and IL-6. Within 2 hours, mRNA for IL-10 appeared following intrapulmonary deposition of immune complexes [20]. Shortly thereafter, IL-10 protein could be detected by Western blot analysis in bronchoalveolar lavage (BAL) fluids and in lung homogenates. The proof that IL-10 was functioning as an endogenous inhibitor was assessed by the use of a blocking antibody to IL-10. When this antibody was instilled intratracheally together with the anti-BSA, significant enhancement of inflammatory injury was noted. Vascular permeability and neutrophil recruitment were each increased by approximately 50%. Accompanying these changes was a significant increase in BAL levels of TNFα. Thus, when endogenous IL-10 is blocked by the presence of antibody, more TNFα is generated, more neutrophils are recruited, and inflammatory injury is accentuated.

Similar findings have been obtained in studies of endogenous IL-6 [19]. During the inflammatory response, IL-6 mRNA and protein were both upregulated. Exogenously administered IL-6 (via the airways) suppressed BAL levels of TNFα, neutrophil accumulation, and lung injury. If rats were treated with blocking antibody to IL-6, more neutrophils were recruited and the injury became worse, these events being associated with higher levels of TNFα in BAL fluids. Thus, in the model employed, IL-6 and IL-10 both endogenously regulate the lung inflammatory response and function to contain the ultimate intensity of inflammatory injury that develops after intrapulmonary deposition of immune complexes.

Suppression of NFκB activation by regulatory ILs

As indicated above, the lung inflammatory model requires generation of TNFα, which is well known to be NFκB-dependent. In order to initiate these studies, nuclear extracts from lung tissues as well as from BAL macrophages were obtained at various time points and analyzed for NFκB content using electrophoretic mobility shift assays (EMSA). This technology utilizes ^{32}P-labeled oligonucleotides containing a sequence identical to the DNA promoter sequence to which NFκB binds. BAL macrophages retrieved within 30 minutes of IgG immune complex deposition showed evidence of NFκB activation (nuclear translocation), while whole lung nuclear extracts did not show maximal NFκB activation until 3-4 hours after the initiation of the inflammatory response [3]. These findings suggested that there may be two waves of NFκB activation in lung, the first affecting macrophages and the second involving different, but as yet unidentified, cell types in the lung. It is quite clear that this process of NFκB activation is both TNFα- and IL-1-dependent, since blocking antibody to either TNFα or IL-1 greatly suppressed intrapulmonary activation of NFκB [3]. Furthermore, intrapulmonary instillation of either TNFα or IL-1, in the absence of any other manipulation, caused lung activation of NFκB. In the immune complex model of lung injury whether TNFα and IL-1 work in sequence or simultaneously to bring about NFκB activation and upregulation of lung vascular ICAM-1 is unknown. As indicated above, IL-10 and IL-13, when exogenously given into lung, suppress TNFα and IL-1 production *in vivo* and greatly diminish the subsequent upregulation of lung vascular ICAM-1 [17, 18].

Our recent studies have been focused on effects of exogenously administered IL-10 or IL-13 on activation of lung NFκB. When 1.0 μg recombinant mouse IL-10 or IL-13 was administered intratracheally with the anti-BSA, it was clear that activation of NFκB in BAL macrophages as well as in whole lung nuclear extracts was suppressed. Supershift electrophoretic assays revealed that, in this inflammatory model, the bulk of NFκB components localizing to nuclei were the p50 and p65 components of NFκB, as opposed to p52, p68 or p75 subunits [3, 22]. The presence of IL-10 or IL-13 interfered with nuclear localization of both subunits of NFκB. A striking observation was the finding by Western blot analysis that, when the lung inflammatory response was triggered in the absence of exogenously administered IL-10 or IL-13, extracts from whole lung and from BAL macrophages revealed a substantial loss of cytoplasmic IκBα during development of the lung inflammatory response [22]. This loss of protein mass is consistent with the expected hydrolysis of IκBα by the 26S proteasome. When inflammatory reactions were carried out in the presence of 1.0 μg IL-10 or IL-13, cytoplasmic levels of IκBα (as determined by Western blot analysis) did *not* undergo that expected loss of mass that was so evident in positive controls which were not otherwise manipulated. Under these conditions, Northern blot analysis failed to reveal any increase in mRNA for p65, suggesting that "preservation" of IκBα levels was not due to transcriptional activation but, rather, was apparently due to protection of IκBα from degradation. Accordingly, it appears that, in the presence of either IL-10 or IL-13, cytoplasmic levels of IκBα are preserved in extracts of whole lungs as well as in extracts of lung macrophages. This is most likely due to the failure of IκBα to be enzymatically broken down, whether because of defective phosphorylation or ubiquination of IκBα, blockade of 26S proteasome activity, inhibition of phosphatases, or other perturbations. This chain of events is reviewed in Fig. 1. Whatever the mechanism, the

Intrapulmonary deposition of IgG immune complexes
↓
Gene activation leading to macrophage expression
of IL-6, IL-10, IL-12, IL-13
↓
Blockade in breakdown of IκBα in the NFκB · IκBα complex
↓
Interference in gene activation of lung macrophages
↓
Suppressed production of TNFα and IL-1
↓
Reduced upregulation of lung vascular ICAM-1
↓
Reduced neutrophil recruitment
↓
Diminished lung injury

Fig. 1. Mechanisms of action of regulatory interleukins

failure of IκBα to be degraded would likely "freeze" NFκB in its inactive state, preventing its translocation into the nucleus and gene activation, which requires the binding of NFκB to promoter sequences on DNA.

The phenomena observed *in vivo* have also been reproduced *in vitro*. When BAL macrophages from normal rat lung were exposed *in vitro* to buffer or to IgG immune complexes, the anticipated activation of NFκB occurred. As expected, loss of IκBα was also noted under conditions of macrophage activation. In the co-presence of either IL-10 or IL-13, no loss of IκBα was demonstrated [22]. Accordingly, it is considered that in isolated macrophages and in lung cells the triggering of the inflammatory response is associated with NFκB activation, which leads to gene activation, the generation of TNFα and by lung macrophages, and IL-1 and the upregulation of vascular adhesion molecules (ICAM-1, E-selectin) that are essential for recruitment of neutrophils. These observations may have implications for therapeutic interventions in humans with inflammatory disorders.

Conclusions

Inflammatory reactions initiated by intrapulmonary deposition of IgG immune complexes are associated with production of TNFα and IL-1, which serve to induce upregulation of vascular adhesion molecules. These cytokines then activate and transcriptionally upregulate vascular endothelial cells followed by the appearance of ICAM-1 and E-selectin, which are essential for neutrophil recruitment. The intensity of these inflammatory reactions is intrinsically limited by anti-inflammatory IL's, such as IL-6 and IL-10, which are expressed in the course of these inflammatory reactions. It has been demonstrated that a common theme of the regulatory IL's is that they suppress intrapulmonary generation of TNFα, reducing lung vascular expression of ICAM-1. The mechanism by which regulatory IL's suppress generation of TNFα appears to be due to interference in NFκB activation. The interference is associated with a retention in cytosolic levels of IκBα, which is ordinarily broken down during cell activation events of the inflammatory response. Retention of IκBα thus prevents the nuclear translocation of NFκB, the consequences of which are a suppressed inflammatory response. These data suggest that interventions which are directed at inhibiting activation of NFκB may represent a useful therapeutic intervention for suppressing the inflammatory response.

References

1. Johnson KJ, Ward PA (1974) Acute immunologic pulmonary alveolitis. J Clin Invest 54: 349-357
2. Lukacs NW, Ward PA (1996) Inflammatory mediators, cytokines, and adhesion molecules in pulmonary inflammation and injury. In: Dixon FJ (ed) Advances in immunology, vol. 62. Academic Press, Orlando, pp 257-304
3. Lentsch AB, Czermak BJ, Bless NM, Ward PA (1998) NF-kB activation during IgG immune complex-induced lung injury. Am J Pathol 152:1327-1336
4. Hugli TE (1986) Biochemistry and biology of anaphylatoxins. Complement 3:111-127
5. Mulligan MS, Vaporciyan AA, Miyasaka M et al (1993) Tumor necrosis factor α regulates in vivo intrapulmonary expression of ICAM-1. Am J Pathol 142:1739-1749
6. Warren JS (1991) Intrapulmonary interleukin 1 mediates acute immune complex alveolitis in the rat. Biochem Biophys Res Commun 175:604-610
7. Mulligan MS, Varani J, Dame MK et al (1991) Role of endothelial-leukocyte adhesion molecule 1 (ELAM-1) in neutrophil-mediated lung injury in rats. J Clin Invest 88:1396-1406
8. Kilgore KS, Shen JP, Miller BF et al (1995) Enhancement by the complement membrane attack complex of tumor necrosis factor-α induced endothelial cell expression of E-selectin and ICAM-1. J Immunol 155:1434-1441
9. Hattori R, Hamilton KK, Fugate RD et al (1998) Stimulated secretion of endothelial von Willebrand factor is accompanied by rapid redistribution to the cell surface of the intracellular granule membrane protein GMP-140. J Biol Chem 264:7768-7771
10. Foreman KE, Vaporciyan AA, Bonish BK et al (1994) C5a-induced expression of P-selectin in endothelial cells. J Clin Invest 94:1147-1155
11. Kilgore KS, Ward PA, Warren JS (1998) Neutrophil adhesion to human endothelial cells is induced by the membrane attack complex: The roles of P-selectin and platelet activating factor. Inflammation (in press)
12. Mulligan MS, Ward PA (1992) Immune complex-induced lung and dermal vascular injury: Differing requirements for TNFα and IL-1. J Immunol 149:331-339
13. Liou HC, Baltimore D (1993) Regulation of the NF-kappa B/rel transcription factor and I kappa B inhibitor system. Curr Opin Cell Biol 5:477-487
14. Baldwin AS (1996) The NF-kappa B and I kappa B proteins: new discoveries and insights. Annu Rev Immunol 14:649-683
15. Kilgore KS, Schmid E, Shanley TP et al (1997) Sublytic concentrations of the membrane attack complex (MAC) of complement induce endothelial interleukin 8 (IL-8) and monocyte protein 1 (MCP-1) through nuclear factor kappa-B (NF-kB) activation. Am J Pathol 150(6): 2019-2031

16. Zimmerman GA, Prescott SM, McIntyre TM (1998) Endothelial cell interactions with granulocytes: tethering and signaling molecules. Immunol Today 13:93-99
17. Mulligan MS, Jones ML, Vaporciyan AA et al (1993) Protective effects of IL-4 and IL-10 against immune complex-induced lung injury. J Immunol 151:5666-5674
18. Mulligan MS, Warner RL, Foreback JL et al (1997) Protective effects of IL-4, IL-10, IL-12, and IL-13 in IgG immune complex-induced lung injury; role of endogenous IL-12. J Immunol 159:3483-3489
19. Shanley TP, Foreback JL, Remick DG et al (1997) Regulatory effects of IL-6 in IgG immune complex-induced lung injury. Am J Pathol 151(1):193-203
20. Shanley TP, Schmal H, Friedl HP et al (1995) Regulatory effects of intrinsic IL-10 in IgG immune complex-induced lung injury. J Immunol 154:3454-3460
21. Schimmer RC, Schrier DJ, Flory CM et al (1998) Streptococcal cell wall-induced arthritis: requirements for IL-4, IL-10, Interferon-γ and MCP-1. J Immunol 160:1466-1471
22. Lentsch AB, Czermak BJ, Bless et al (1998) NF-kB activation during IgG immune complex-induced lung injury: requirements for TNFα and IL-1β but not complement. Am J Pathol 152:1327-1336

CLINICAL INTERVENTIONS
IN THE FIELD OF SEPSIS

WHAT IS WRONG AND WHAT IS RIGHT

Shall We Continue to Talk About (or Use) SIRS in the Twenty-first Century?

J.-L. VINCENT

Sepsis is a frequent cause of death on our intensive care units (ICUs) and despite advances in our understanding of the processes involved and elucidation of the inflammatory cascade, we remain no closer to finding a cure. The terminology employed in discussing disease processes is often confusing and frequently inadequate, perhaps never more so than with regard to the septic patient. Many words and phrases have been, and are, used in an attempt to define and describe the septic patient, including "infection", "bacteraemia", "septicaemia", "severe sepsis", "sepsis syndrome" [1].

The word "sepsis" is derived from a Greek word meaning putrefaction and in present usage could in fact be defined as being the host response to infection [2]. The word "infection" implies the presence of an invading microorganism whether of viral, fungal or bacterial origin. In response to infection, the body puts in motion a complex inflammatory response in an attempt to eradicate the offending organism. It is this reaction which creates the classical clinical, haemodynamic and biochemical picture of sepsis. However, the same reaction may occur in conditions in which no infection can be demonstrated such as acute pancreatitis, trauma, ischaemia/reperfusion or even severe heart failure.

In order to categorize such processes, the term systemic inflammatory response syndrome (SIRS) was proposed by a consensus conference of the American College of Chest Physicians and the Society of Critical Care Medicine in 1991 [3]. SIRS was thus introduced in an attempt to simplify current confusion, and as a concept is well-intentioned. Using the terminology proposed by this consensus conference [3], sepsis is now defined as SIRS associated with a confirmed infection, severe sepsis as sepsis with organ dysfunction, hypotension or evidence of hypoperfusion, and septic shock as sepsis with hypotension and hypoperfusion. The suggestion is that there is a hierarchical continuum from SIRS through sepsis to septic shock [3], and several studies have confirmed that this does indeed appear to occur [4-6]. As patients progress along this continuum from SIRS to septic shock, they, perhaps not unexpectedly, experience worsening organ function and increased mortality. In a study by Rangel-Frausto et al. [4], involving 3708 patients from ICUs and general wards, 68% of all patients met the SIRS criteria. Of these, 26% developed sepsis, 18% severe sepsis and 4% septic shock. In the progression from SIRS increasing proportions of patients had acute respiratory distress syndrome (ARDS), disseminated intravascular coagulation (DIC) and acute renal failure. The mortality rate associated with a diagnosis of SIRS was 7%, rising to 16% for sepsis, 20% for severe sepsis and 46% for septic shock. Similarly, Salvo et al. [5] studied 1101 ICU patients and found that 58% fulfilled SIRS criteria at some point during their stay. Mortality rates again increased with the clinical progression from SIRS to septic shock, 26.5% in SIRS, 36% in sepsis, 52.2% in severe sepsis and 81.8% in septic shock. Another study [7] on patients admitted to general medical wards who had blood taken for culture, found that 55% of patients fulfilled SIRS criteria and SIRS patients had a mortality rate of 36% compared to 38% for patients with severe sepsis and 56% for septic shock. In a further study [6] in ICU patients, the length of ICU stay, as well as the mortality rate, was shown to increase as patients progressed from a diagnosis of SIRS to severe sepsis.

Several studies [4-6] thus support the concept of a clinical progression from SIRS to septic shock, associated with increased complications and worsened outcome. However, SIRS has several shortcomings [8], and rather than clarify the "sepsis" issue, the use of this term adds further confusion.

The problems with SIRS

1. We already have many terms to describe "sepsis" and do not really need any more. We should come to some agreement of how and when to use the phrases already available before we add others. In fact, the words infection and sepsis are too frequently used as direct synonyms and we should be clearer in our use of "infection" to indicate the presence of an invading microorganism, and "sepsis" to indicate the inflammatory response to that organism. The clinician understands that saying someone "looks septic", does not mean the same as saying someone is "infected". Admittedly it is not always easy to recognize or demonstrate an infection in critically ill patients, many of whom will already be receiving antibiotics. Employing the term SIRS for such patients may reduce the incentive to search aggressively for infection, with serious consequences.

2. The definition of SIRS as proposed by the consensus conference [3] are much too sensitive. SIRS criteria are met by the acute change from baseline of two or more of the following parameters: fever ($>38°C$) or hypothermia ($<36°C$); tachycardia (heart rate >90 beats/min); tachypnoea (respiratory rate >20 breaths/min) or hyperventilation ($PaCO_2 <30$ mmHg or <4.3 kPa); white blood cell count >12000 cells/mm^3 or <4000 cells/mm^3. As we have seen, a large percentage of ICU patients [4-6] and many general ward patients [4, 7] meet these criteria. Indeed, using data from the SOFA database [9], and analyzing a subgroup of patients who stayed on the ICU for at least one week, we have observed that all the patients in this subgroup met the

SIRS criteria at some point (unpublished data). SIRS could thus be said to be a synonym for "critically ill patient".

3. SIRS criteria can be used by clinical researchers as inclusion criteria for patient entry to clinical trials, with the support of a consensus conference. However, as we have seen, SIRS can be applied to many critically ill patients and such trials will therefore be conducted on a very non-specific group of patients. We have already seen the limitations of studies based on heterogeneous groups of patients with the many negative trials of sepsis treatments (Table 1), although many of these agents may in fact be of benefit in certain selected groups of patients [10]. We may have dismissed potentially effective drugs on the grounds that we could not show that they worked, yet with more selective patient inclusion criteria, perhaps we would have had more positive results. The use of SIRS as an inclusion criteria will not be of help in identifying those patients who may benefit most from new therapies.

Table 1. Immunomodulating strategies tested in clinical trials with negative results

Monoclonal antibodies to lipid A: HA1A, E5
Anti-tumor necrosis factor (TNF) antibodies
TNF soluble receptors (p 55 and p 75)
Interleukin-1 receptor antagonist
Platelet activating factor (PAF) antagonists
Corticosteroids
Ibuprofen
Ketoconazole
Thromboxane synthetase inhibitors
Prostaglandin (PGE$_1$)
Nitric oxide (NO) synthase inhibitors

Conclusions

I am afraid that in spite of the drawbacks and potentially harmful aspects of SIRS discussed above, the term, SIRS, will continue to be used, by some, in the 21st century. This is largely because the underlying concept is sound, and the idea is simple. However, medicine is never simple and SIRS oversimplifies what is a very complex phenomenon. We must acknowledge that our understanding of sepsis and the inflammatory cascade of mediators has improved greatly in recent years, but much remains unknown. Further study is indeed necessary to unravel all the complexities of sepsis before we will be able to identify which agents will be effective in which groups of patients. Clearly, clinical trials will no longer simply start from the SIRS criteria, but will need to employ a more selective approach to patient entry. Our approach to endpoints also needs to alter with outcomes focusing on morbidity as well as mortality [11]. Sepsis is a complicated process but the terminology associated with it need not be, we have sufficient words without needing to introduce new ones. Playing with words is of no benefit to us or our patients: the search for an effective immunomodulating strategy remains our great challenge.

References

1. Balk RA, Bone RC (1989) The septic syndrome: Definition and clinical implications. Crit Care Clin 5:1-8
2. Vincent JL (1994) Sepsis and septic shock: Update on definitions. In: Reinhart K, Eyrich K, Sprung C (eds) Sepsis: Current perspectives in pathophysiology and therapy. Springer, Berlin Heidelberg New York, pp 3-15
3. Members of the American College of Chest Physicians/Society of Critical Care Medicine Consensus Conference Committee (1992) Definitions for sepsis and organ failure and guidelines for the use of innovative therapies in sepsis. Crit Care Med 20:864-874
4. Rangel-Frausto MS, Pittet D, Costigan M et al (1995) The natural history of the systemic inflammatory response syndrome (SIRS). A prospective study. JAMA 273:117-123
5. Salvo I, de Cian W, Musicco M et al (1995) The Italian SEPSIS study: Preliminary results on the incidence and evolution of SIRS, sepsis, severe sepsis and septic shock. Intensive Care Med 21:S244-S249
6. Pittet D, Rangel-Frausto S, Li N et al (1995) Systemic inflammatory response syndrome, sepsis, severe sepsis and septic shock: incidence, morbidities and outcomes in surgical patients. Intensive Care Med 21:302-309
7. Jones GR, Lowes JA (1996) The systemic inflammatory response syndrome as a predictor of bacteremia and outcome from sepsis. QJM 89:515-522
8. Vincent JL (1997) Dear SIRS, I'm sorry to say I don't like you. Crit Care Med 25:372-374
9. Vincent JL, Moreno R, Takala J et al (1996) The SOFA (sepsis-related organ failure assessment) score to describe organ dysfunction/failure. Intensive Care Med 22:707-710
10. Vincent JL (1998) Sepsis: The search continues for effective immunomodulating strategies. Lancet 351:922-923
11. Vincent JL (1997) New therapies in sepsis. Chest 112:330S-338S

Prevention and Treatment of Sepsis - Present and Future Problems

A.E. Baue

What is wrong is that we have become lumpers – lumping together various human illnesses and injuries and attempting to treat them based upon certain general symptoms (SIRS, for example). This approach has not worked nor will it. What is right is that we are beginning to recognize this and we are becoming splitters. The evolution of Roger Bones thinking about this is worth reviewing. Early on he was excited about SIRS and MODS and developed concepts of CARS, MARS, and CHAOS [1]. As more and more magic bullets failed, he progressively stressed the need to break down into separate units the problems you deal with within an ICU. From a lumper he was becoming a splitter. The day is over, or should be, when we attempt to treat a group of symptoms or signs which simply indicate that the patient is sick. This approach does not work.

I will emphasize five points in my further discussion: 1) Curing the disease, or reducing mortality requires specific therapy for the cause of that disease; 2) This is not the first time when salient therapeutic prospects from the experimental laboratory have been unsuccessful in patients; 3) The problems of lumpers and splitters – do we divide the trials into separate disease categories? Do we lump them altogether with some nonspecific entry criteria?; 4) Present and future problems: a) harbingers of doom and b) biologic conundrums; 5) The future lies ahead – where do we go ahead from here? We must also consider risk factors and the possibility of multi-agent therapy.

Curing a disease requires specific therapy

There have been magic bullets in the past and they have all been directed toward or against a specific disease or a specific category of therapy [2], I have reviewed this in my paper on relevance. After so many potential magic bullets for SIRS, sepsis, or inflamed patients have failed in the recent past, many drug companies have pulled back their efforts and focused on specific diseases of inflammation such as rheumatoid arthritis. There are three clinical trials of anti-inflammatory agents to try to control this disease (Table 1).

Table 1. Rheumatoid arthritis (a specific inflammatory disease)

TNFR:Fcp80	A fusion protein for human soluble TNF receptors (Immunex)
IDEC-CD 91	An anti-CD 4 monoclonal antibody (IDEC Company)
rhIL-Ira	IL-1 receptor antagonist (AMGEN Company)

All of these agents quiet down the inflammatory process
Phase II trials are very encouraging
Will they prevent joint destruction?

These studies are very encouraging in phase II trials. All the studies quiet down the inflammatory process in patients. The question that requires time and an eventual answer is: "Will these agents prevent joint destruction?" [3]. This work excites me. It is direct and specifically directed against a disease which is known to be due to inflammatory mediators. At the present time anti-inflammatory agents do not cure any diseases or injuries. If they ever do, it will be a pure inflammatory disease. They decrease or modulate inflammation and, therefore, may decrease symptoms and make you feel better – take the edge off.

As I have written earlier, Stehben, a pathologist in New Zealand, has urged us to focus on the cause of a disease. He states that "It is essential to differentiate between specific diseases and those conditions which represent a class of disorders, complications common to many diseases and merely symptoms, signs, a physical state or laboratory findings" [4]. "Treatment of a disease, when based on symptoms or clinical manifestations, is at best palliative and nonspecific". Aspirin for the flu may make you feel better but it does nothing for the underlying disease. This is exemplified by therapeutic efforts to treat SIRS. What would you do? The possibilities are shown in Table 2. Obviously this is ridiculous. I hope it makes the point that you cannot treat SIRS. You must treat the underlying disease or injury. Thus, using SIRS as the entry criterion for a trial of a therapeutic agent is doomed to failure.

Table 2. Early treatment of SIRS

1. Temperature
   a) If low, warm patient with warming blankets, extracorporeal warming circuit, warm i.v. fluids, irrigate peritoneal cavity with warm saline
   b) If high, use external cooling, cool bath, rectal aspirin, etc.
2. Rapid heart rate - slow with calcium channel blockade, rapid-acting digitalis, etc.
3. Rapid breathing - i.v. morphine, other sedation, intubation, paralysis and controlled ventilation
4. For low WBC - give G-CSF
   For a high WBC - consider chemotherapeutic agents to control the blood marrow

SIRS, systemic inflammatory response syndrome

We tend to lump sick patients together in various classifications or categories, based on severity, the possibility of death, clinical manifestations, ICU admissions, and other criteria such as APACHE, SAPS, SIRS, MODS, MOF and ISS. If such classifications of patients are used as the entry criteria for therapy trials, we may miss important treatments. Some therapies may be excellent in certain diseases or abnormalities and worthless in others even though the disease severity may be similar in both.

There have been many previous unsuccessful therapeutic efforts
History is a valuable teacher

There have been many agents that were exciting in the animal laboratory and many of us studied them extensively but they never made it into clinical use or survived clinical trials [5]. There were exciting moments in the laboratory where we thought they had specific effects. I will give examples of these in the paper on clinical relevance.

Careful controlled studies of various treatment modalities in normal animals with one perturbation (i.e. haemorrhage, cecal ligation and puncture (CLP), *E. coli* infusion and endotoxin infusion) or two perturbations, haemorrhage plus fracture, burn plus CLP, and therapy may yield statistically significant positive results but the results may be clinically irrelevant.

The major reasons for this are variations in human disease such as the following: 1) The disease process – what is it? Pancreatitis is different from perforated diverticulitis and both differ from the adult respiratory distress syndrome; 2) severity of disease; 3) extent of disease; 4) duration of disease; 5) remote organ function and chronic health problems; 6) age of the patient; 7) genetic differences and responses of the individual; 8) complications; 9) therapy – time and dose, duration; 10) other therapy or organ support. Also, some clinical advances seem to initially contribute to better patient care and then fall into disuse simply because they did not make enough difference. They are not worth the trouble.

The problems of lumpers and splitters

Next I will consider the problem of lumpers and splitters which were referred to earlier. Again, history will help us. Pauline Mazumdar, in a new book on the history of immunology, makes a general observation that scientific thinkers or natural philosophers, as they were once called, seemed to be a genus of two species: one genus seeks unity and the other genus distinct categories [6]. In Table 3 one can see where one group seeks unity, continuity, and simplicity in nature. They are unifiers or lumpers. The other group seeks discontinuity, pluralistic approaches, specific abnormalities, and they can be called splitters. This table is adapted from a book review by Lesch [7].

Table 3. Scientific thinkers - Natural philosophers? A genus of two species

One seeks	The other seeks
Unity	Discontinuity
Continuity	Distinct categories
Simplicity in nature	Pluralist
Unifiers	Specific abnormalities
They are Lumpers	They are Splitters

From a book review of Mazumdar by Lesch (modified)

The history of this is shown in Table 4 where scientists tended to separate themselves into these two categories. Obviously there is overlap and some inconsistencies. For example, Landsteiner was a student of von Gruber. They sought unity but Landsteiner described separate blood types.

Table 4. The shaping of modern biology

Group one	Group two
Galileo	Aristotle
Buffon	Linnaeus
Mathias Schleidon (cell theory)	Ferdinand Ohn (bacterial types)
Carl von Nageli	Robert Koch
Max von Gruber	Paul Ehrlich
Karl Landsteiner	Ronald Fisher
Alexander Wiener	Robert Race
Lumpers	**Splitters**

As we move from the twentieth to the twenty-first century we must recognize lumpers and splitters according to their biologic predilections (Table 5). Thus, intensivists, by their specialty, tend to be lumpers instead of splitters because their specialty is support, not specific therapy. They treat all who come to an ICU and they treat critically ill patients. Thus, they treat the critically ill, not specific diseases. There are differences between intensivists, surgeons, physicians, pediatricians, and others. Surgeons must be splitters – operating on specific abnormalities. This is where the selection of general criteria for clinical trials has come a cropper.

Table 5. 20th-21st Centuries

Lumpers	Splitters
Intensivists	Surgeons
SIRS	Separate injuries and diseases
MODS	
Magic bullets	MOF

MODS, multi-organ dysfunction syndrome
MOF, multi-organ failure

Present and future problems

There are several dilemmas we have in our work today. One is with the abnormal factors or values that can be measured in ICU patients which predict an unfavorable outcome. Correcting those abnormalities may not improve mortality. Thus, are they mediators or are they markers? I call these predictors or harbingers of doom. Secondly, there are many examples of mediators which are harmful in some settings but necessary in others. I have called those biological puzzles or conundrums.

Harbingers of doom - Critical event or measurement scoring that predicts disaster (or MOF or ARDS)

"It Ain't Over Until It's Over"

Yogi Berra

A frequent exercise in the ICU is to seek measurements, laboratory tests or pathophysiologic states which predict big trouble, a fatal outcome or both. There are many scoring systems which indicate the severity of illness, or injury and predict the statistical possibilities of death or survival. These include: ISS, Apache I, II and III, MODs score, SOFA, SAPS, LODs and many others.

Many mediator levels, laboratory measurements and other phenomena have been used to suggest a bad outcome (Table 6). None of these scores or tests or levels is accurate enough to use in an individual patient in order to discontinue therapy. We always give the patients the benefit of the doubt in trying for survival even though the odds are bad. Seemingly miraculous recoveries do occur. There are few absolutes in human biology. The Harvard law of experimentation states that: "Under controlled conditions animals and people behave as they damn well please". There are a few conditions that are definitive. As my friend, Father Kevin O'Rourke, states "If your brain is dead, you are dead". Short of that, caring for an ICU patient is always worth a shot. I rely on the progression of events to advise families, friends and the clergy. Progressive deterioration in organ function over some days with no response to therapy with no remedial problem evident is the best indication that the situation is becoming irreversible.

Table 6. Harbingers of doom

Marker or event	Associated with or an ↑ frequency of
Thrombocytopenia	Associated with MOF - Hirasawa
Platelet trapping, sequestration in lungs, liver and gut	Sepsis, MOF - Sigurdsson
↑ soluble thrombomodulin and neutrophil elastase	DIC and MODS - Gando
Serial Lactate-High initially and stays high	MOF - Bakker, Vincent
Initial AT III level with DIC	Predicts death - Fourrier
↑ serum lipofuscin formed from lipid peroxidation	↑ ARDS & MOF - Roumen, et al.
sICAM-1 and sELAM-1	Higher in non-survivor, ↓ in survivors Boldt et al.
↑ adrenomedullin	May contribute to septic shock
↑ pre-op CRP	Predicts post-op complications
Before secondary operation ↑ Neutrophil Elastase, ↑ C reactive protein and ↓ platelet count	Predict organ failure with secondary operations for trauma - Nast-Kolb, Waydhas
Plasma sTNFR p55 and p75 ↑ with sepsis p55 values higher in non-survivors	Sepsis syndrome and death Calvano, Lowre
↑ sTNFR p55	Sepsis and death after cardiac surgery - Pilz
↑ IL-6 in burns	Bacterial sepsis
↑ IL-6 levels early >1000 pg/Ml	Correlates with complications and mortality - Biffl, Moores, et al.
↑ Carboxy haemoglobin	With sepsis - Moncure
Membrane TNFα/TNFR ratio	Correlates with MOD score and death Pellegrini, Carol Miller
IL-8 circulating and in lung fluid ↑ second peck	Larger burns sepsis - ARDS Vinderes, et al. Miller, et al.
Monocyte CD14 expression and HLA-DR exp	Indicates clinical outcome after injury Heinzelman, Cheadle, Polk
Age > 55, ISS > 25, > CuRBCs/12 hour base def - lactate, platelets	Predicted MOF after injury - Sauaia, et al.
↑ IL-6, IL-8, and SICAM-1 early after trauma later ↑	MOF - Patrick, Moores, et al.
Ig MendoCab ↓ (anti-endotoxin core antibody)	Predicted poor post-op outcome after cardiac surg Duke University - Bennett Guerrero
Number of blood transfusions after injury	MOF - Moore
Group II PLA₂	Lethal MOF in patients with injuries or diffuse peritonitis - Nyman
Procalcitonin ↑	Sepsis Assicot
Neutrophil elastase, ↑ lactate, antithromb IL-1 ↓ IL-6 and 8 ↑	OF and death - Nast-Kolb
↓ serum IL-1 activity and ↓ monocyte IL-product?	Fatal sepsis - Lugeret, et al.
Low IL-1 in burns and trauma patients bad terminal C3a compl activity and thromboxane Celastase ↑ neopterin/creatinine ratio ↑ later	MOF - Roumen, et al.
Hypothermia	Fatal with sepsis syndrome - Clemmer, et al.
High C-3 terminal complement and thromboxane	Predicts MOF

Outcome Predictive Score	Predicts MOF
↓ ability of patients serum to opsonize heat killed bacteria	
↓ Class II major histocompatibility antigen expression (HLA-DR on peripheral leukocytes)	
IL-10 ↑	Predicts sepsis in trauma patients
Abnormal lactate/pyruvate ratio	Predicts MOF
Human leukocyte antigen (HLA-DR) CD 14 expression - ↓ serum IL-1 and ↓ monocyte IL-1	Correlates with infection and death fatal sepsis, in injured patients
↑ neutrophil elastase, ↑ C-reactive protein ↓ platelet count	
Thrombocytopenia	
↑ sTNFR-55	
Arterial Blood Ketone Body	Dead
Ratio HBKBR < 0.25	
Critical Level 0.4 to 0.25	MOF
Lung, Liver, GI Bleed, Kidney, Cerebral	Ozawa
F. Coagulopathy	
↓ Protein C	Pro-coagulant sepsis and shock
↓ PAF - acetyl hydrolase activity	MOF in trauma patients - Patrick, Moore
↑ B - endorphin	Head injury patients that died Lehmann-Regel
Hypothermia, Neutropenia, shock, MOF, ARDS	Indicate mortality - Balk, Parillo
↓ IGF-1, IGF-IL and IGF bonding protein 3	Critical illness - Timmers, et al.
Plasma erythropoietin and IL-6 ↑	Critically in children - Jacobs
↑ serum C18 unsaturated free fatty acids	ARDS
Cellular injury score (CIS)	MOF - Hirasawa
A refined Apache III including GCS and trauma diagnosis	Predicted mortality
24 hour IC point system with PaO_2/FiO_2 index, GCS and fluid balance	Predicted death
Rapid bedside assay for endotoxin	MODS
Intramucosal pH of sigmoid colon	Acidosis → death in AAA ops
Low monocyte TNFR	Predicted death from sepsis - Barie
Low plasma anti-oxidant potential and does not come up	Unfavorable outcome - Cowley

Is there any value then in listing, describing or reviewing factors that suggest a poor outcome? The levels or factors may have nothing to do with the outcome but are simply markers of severe illness. I believe there is value in such a review (otherwise I would not be writing this) because it helps to define the pathophysiologic events and limits in human disease. Out of this may come an idea, a therapy, or a research project which will increase our understanding. Some factors predict specific abnormalities such as the Adult Respiratory Distress Syndrome (ARDS) and may suggest earlier or alternative therapies. The question really is, are they markers or mediators or both? Further understanding of these agents will come.

Biologic conundrums with serious inflammation due to illness and injury

"A paradox, a paradox, a most ingenious paradox"

Gilbert and Sullivan
The Pirates of Penzance

In a special article in Critical Care Medicine Roger Bone lists a number of conditions that have been associated with increased cytokine levels [8]. This list seems on initial glance as a potpourri of human abnormalities. However, as one contemplates the underlying pathophysiologic mechanisms of items on this list, they are: inflammation due to infection, ischaemia, tissue injury, cell necrosis, or injury. There are some abnormalities where cytokines are said to have been elevated which may fall outside of these categories, but still could have an inflammatory component. These are: a) diabetes; b) advanced age – where apoptosis may be a factor; c) certain tumors, and d) osteoporosis. Also the extent of cytokine involvement with these diseases was not described. Bone raises the question in his conclusions, "Does SIRS represent an evolutionary mechanism to kill off an organism when local wound and infection control have failed?". This could be called organismal apoptosis. I offer an alternative explanation for this conclusion of Bone's and that is that these biologic systems developed or exist to provide for survival of the individual from a maximal insult (injury or infection) without therapy. When the insult is overwhelming, the inflammatory response may also be excessive and no longer protective, but rather a destructive phenomenon (the horror autotoxicus) [9]. This occurs particularly if modern therapy cannot control the injury or infection and thus the excessive inflammation. Thus, it is not a matter of organismal apoptosis, but rather a matter of overwhelming injury and illness which cannot be controlled by our biologic defense systems. We were not designed or did not evolve to survive certain overwhelming injuries or diseases. At the turn of the 20th century, a fractured femur alone was fatal because of bleeding into the thigh muscles. Now multi-system injury, infection and severe inflammatory diseases mark the limits of our therapy and organ support. These defense systems then get out of hand.

A number of cytokines have been thought to be primary mediators of the inflammatory response leading to SIRS, MODS and MOF. Substantial evidence has been gathered for this by infusion of cytokines, such as TNFα, IL-1β, endotoxin and other mediators in animals and human volunteers, and by blockade of such cytokines by monoclonal antibodies before infusion of endotoxin, gramnegative bacteria or other substances [10]. However, inflammation involves many processes in addition to cytokines, such as complement, the autocoids, and kallikreins, growth factors, polymorphonuclear leukocytes releasing proteases and oxygen radicals, T-cells, B-cells, and others [11]. Cytokines are also very necessary factors to heal wounds, fight infection, and control tissue injury. In certain disease processes, cytokines seem necessary or at least blockade of their effects leads to increased mortality or extent of injury (Table 7). Examples include the use of an anti-TNF mab which increases mortality in experimental peritonitis [12]. High TNF serum levels are associated with increased survival in patients with abdominal septic shock [13]. Administration of IL-1 and indomethacin to burned mice with peritonitis improved survival [14]. Low circulating IL-1 concentrations have been associated with increased mortality in burned patients [15]. IL-1β given to mice improves survival after cecal ligation and puncture [16]. High levels of IL-6 are associated with increased mortality in many abnormalities [17, 18]. However, IL-6, when injected into animals, produces only lymph node hyperplasia [18]. IL-1α prevents lethality in *E. Coli* [19] peritonitis and protects animals against endotoxin [20]. Low IL-1 is a negative predictor for fatal sepsis in patients [21]. Mast cells are detrimental in allergic reactions and are protective in some infections [22]. Finally, IL-10 protects mice during septic peritonitis [23] but neutralization of IL-10 increases survival in *Klebsiella* pneumonia [24].

Table 7. Biologic conundrums

TNF and IL-1 KO mice	Resistant to endotoxin
only IL-1 KO	Resistant to *E. Coli* peritonitis
TNF deficient c3H/HcJ mice but	↑ survival from haemorrhagic shock
anti-TNF mab →	Abolished ↑ TNF but did not ↑ survival
TNF mab	Protects against endotoxin infusion but increases mortality with CLP
High TNF levels	Associated with survival in patients with abdominal septic shock
IL-1β and TNFα	- ↑ with endotoxin in human volunteers but levels do not correlate in sick patients, IL-1β levels correlated with survival TNFα correlated with severity
Macrophage deficient mice → (absent CSF-1)	↓ TNF, IL-1, GCSF and endotoxin induced bacterial translocation but morbidity and mortality same as in normal animals
TNFα p80R (Fc fusion protein)	↓ bioactive TNFα in neutropenic, i.v. *E. Coli* rats but no effect on lung injury or mortality
TNFα	1. necessary for liver hepatic regeneration 2. produces inflammation in the liver
Lactated Ringers	↑ cytokine release IL-2, IL-6, IL-10 TNFα with or without haemorrhage
Cytokines (IL-8, TNFα IL-1β)	Enhance PMN bactericidal activity Receptor binding ↓ resistance to infection
Germ-free animals after haemorrhagic shock	Have increased survival but increased inflammatory mediators
TNF	Produces focal ischaemic brain damage
TNFr KO	Cerebral ischaemic damage ↑
Partial liquid ventilation (perflubron)	Protects lungs but ↑ TNF in BAL
TNF	Enhances antibiotic efficacy after haemorrhagic shock
IL-1ra in patients	↑ IL-1 ↑ LTB$_4$ ↓ T$_x$B$_2$, PGI Leukotrienes TNF and IL-6
rhIL-1a	↑ resistance to bacterial infection

Abscess model	Anorexia, weight loss and hepatic-acute phase response is due in part to IL binding to type I receptor
	TNF binding is not required
IL-1	Produces catabolism protein, anorexia, fever weight loss
Haemorrhage	Protected against LPS + IL-1ICE - greater protection attenuates IL-1
IL-6 deficient mice with liver failure	Have defective hepatocyte reg
Anti-IL-6 mab given to endotoxemic mice	Yields increased IL-6
Interferon γ given to normal animals	Increased the response to LPS and increased lethality of bacteria/challenge
Interferon γ	Primes only a subpopulation of PMNS (leukocytes)
Interferon γ - deficient mice	Die of infection but if given to animals after injury decreased lethal abdominal sepsis
CLP-anti-IL-10	All die
CLP + IL-10-survival ↑	
IL-10	Anti-IL-10 ↑ survival with K pneumonia
	Endogenous IL-10 protects from CLP
	Anti-IL-10 restores T-cell function in burns
	IL-10 contributes to post-injury immunodepression
	IL-10 ↓ endotoxin induced cytokines
	rhIL-10 proposed for aneurysm operations
	IL-10 KO die of inflammation not infection
PAF antagonist	- ↑ mortality after trauma in swine
	↓ mortality to LPS
LPS pretreatment	Protects lungs from hepatic ischaemia/reperfusion
LPS →	Induces PGE2 which ↓ macrophage
	TNF production
PAF	Primes PMNs for superoxides and elastase release
PAF antagonist	↑ mortality after trauma and haemorrhage
	↓ mortality in swine to LPS
β-adrenergic stim.	Inhibit PAF superoxide priming but not elastase release
Polymyxin decreased plasma endotoxin levels	But there was no decrease in sepsis scores, IL-6 or mortality
Recombinant tissue plasminogen activator	Decreases abscesses in rats with peritonitis but increases bacteraemia and death
Glutathione	The most abundant intracellular anti-oxidant
Glutathione depletion (diethyl maleate)	↑ survival after cerebral I/R
	↓ liver injury from endotoxin
	↓ lung injury
	↓ LPS skin inflammation
Macrophage depleted mice	↑ systemic bacterial translocation
	↓ systemic toxic response
	↓ mortality
Intestinal permeability is increased by trauma and shock	But there is no relation to septic complications
L-arginine	Required for normal lymphocyte proliferation, pharmacologic doses inhibit proliferation
Immune-enhancing patients diet in trauma	Exaggerated immune response and increased ARDS

Complement inhibition	↓ inflammation
	↓ I/R injury
	but
	↓ host defense
Neutrophils CLP	Anti-CD 18 rx
	↑ remote organ neutrophil sequestration in the liver and lung and
	↑ liver injury
Inhibition of CD 11/18 (mab) - integrin receptor on neutrophils	with intrabronchial E. coli improved lung function but ↑ mortality
Anti-adhesion molecules	Protect endothelium and microvasculature
	↑ infection
CD11/18 mab with intra-bronchial E. Coli	↓ lung neutrophils
	↑ lung function
	↑ mortality
CD 11/18 mab	↑ survival with TNF challenge
A leukocyte CD18 mab	Increases endotoxaemia and CV injury with septic shock
Selection blockade	↑ LPS induced lung injury
PGE$_2$	Produces immunosuppression
but	
rats - 30% body	Ibuprofen ↓ certain aspects of immune function
but	
rats - CLP	Ibuprofen ↓ survival
Ibuprofen	↑ mortality in vivo of CLP in rats, in vitro PGE inhibits multiple leukocyte functions and Ibuprofen blocks that. PGE prevents excessive product of TNF
Indomethacin	In vivo and in vitro do not correlate ↕ different
	↑ mortality with endotoxaemia
	↓ mortality with burn/sepsis CLP stopped two days before
PGE$_2$	Helps the liver respond to inflammatory stimuli
	contributes to immunosuppression
NSAIDS	Protect against endotoxaemia
	but ↑ TNF production
Angiopoieton (Ang-1)	Endo cell specific
	Tie 2 receptors
	tyrosine kinase
	Required for tissue repair
	Tumors subvert
Prophylactic G-CSF upregulates → immune response ↑ neutrophil function - with filgrastin	May improve or worsen organ failure
Transforming growth factor TGF-B	– beneficial effect on wound healing
	– is a key factor in fibrogenesis
Ang-2	A natural antagonist
	Expressed at sites
	Of vascular remodeling
	? needed to control wound repair
TGF-B	Initiates and terminates tissue repair but sustained production ↑ fibrogenesis - tissue fibrosis
rhGH in burns	↑ constitutive protein synthesis
	↓ hepatocyte growth factors (HGF)

Major torso trauma	Colony stimulating activity ↓
	Inadequate granulopoiesis
Glucocorticoids	Induce MIF (macrophage migration inhibitory factor)
	MIF - counters the immunosuppression of steroids
Marmoset model of multiple	Marmoscles tolerized to MOG did not get MS - but a lethal
sclerosis - produced by MOG	demyelinating disorder developed
myelin oligodendrocyte	T cells shifted from T_H2 pattern. Immune deviation can increase
glycoprotein	pathogenic auto-antibodies
NF - KB nuclear factor	↑ gene expression for mediators of chronic inflammatory
Inflammatory diseases	diseases
	blockade may ↓ manifestation of chronic inflammatory diseases
	But 1. Knockout of p65 comp of NF-KB is lethal
	But 2. lack of p50 - produces immune def and
	↑ susceptibility to infection
Partial liquid ventilation	Lung protective but ↑ BAL TNF
Blockage of inflammatory	Can have a positive or a negative effect
mediators	

Brett Giroir has said that we have become too focused on the toxic effects of cytokines rather than on their functions in health. Thus, there are many biologic conundrums or puzzles that present a challenge to us. Too much pro-inflammation – or too little; too much anti-inflammation or too little – differences in isolated organ ischaemia/reperfusion and whole body ischaemia – shock.

The question quite simply is will further definition of a generalized biologic problem SIRS, MODS, MOF, CARS, CHAOS contribute to reduced morbidity and mortality or should we rather focus on specific disease processes and their manifestations – pro- and anti-inflammatory manifestation and mechanisms of organ injury and death? I vote for disease specific studies and therapy. A number of these biologic conundrums or puzzles are listed in Table 7. They could also be called ambiguities.

The future lies ahead

Where do we go from here? If we review risk factors for sepsis, complications and extent of injury, we find out we have had very little control over them. Age, the Apache score, the injury severity score, days in the ICU, amount of blood loss with injury or operation, chronic diseases such as heart disease, COPD, chronic renal failure are all predetermined. Some may be preventable before the insult and this requires emphasis.

Multi-agent therapy may be required and I have discussed this in detail in an accompanying paper.

Finally, what is sepsis? Is it a valuable concept? How do you treat sepsis? – properly, correctly, successfully but with what? I know well the development of the terms beginning with infection, to bacteraemia, septicaemia, sepsis and sepsis syndrome and finally to SIRS and MODS. What have we gained? With infection – what kind? – what organisms? Pneumonia, peritonitis, abscess, cellulitis, wound infection, emphysema, pericarditis, cholangitis, hepatitis, endotoxaemia – all differ from each other and they differ from tissue injury – tissue necrosis and inflammation such as pancreatitis.

One of our problems is that ICUs become bacteriologic cesspools. Catheters and tubes and wounds and the gut are constant sources of infection. Christou et al. cite the constant exposure to contamination in the ICU and suggests that this is the reason why overall ICU mortality has not changed [25]. Avoiding an ICU may be beneficial. Thus, we again come to prevention – prevention of injury – prevention of complications – prevention of infection and then organ support to prevent failure [26]. Our problems present and future are listed in Table 8.

Table 8. Problems - Present and future

1.	Harbingers of doom	Causes or indicators?
2.	Biologic conundrums	Too little is lethal, too much is a disaster
3.	Early diagnosis	Is it early enough?
4.	Immunobiologic variability	on seemingly similar patient
5.	Male or female	With overwhelming injury there is a difference
6.	Integrative non-linear biology	There seems to be no homeostasis but rather dyshomeostasis overwhelming injury

References

1. Bone RC (1996) Sir Isaac Newton, sepsis, SIRS and CARS. Crit Care Med 24:1125-1138
2. Baue AE (1997) Multiple Organ Failure, Multiple Organ Dysfunction Syndrome and Systemic Inflammatory Response Syndrome - Why no magic bullets? Arch Surg 132:703-707
3. Skolnick AA (1997) Biological response modifiers may yield a new class of drugs to treat arthritis. JAMA 277:276-278
4. Stehben WE (1993) Causality in medical science with particular reference to heart disease and arteriosclerosis. Persp Biol Med 36:97-119
5. Baue AE (1983) Shock research and therapy in the 1980's. Keynote address. In: SM Reichard and RR Wolfe (eds). Advances in Shock Research 4:1-16
6. Mazumdar PMH (1995) Species and specificity: an interpretation of the history of immunology. Science xiv:457, Cambridge University Press, New York
7. Lesch JE (1996) Immunology dichotomized. 273:75-76
8. Bone RL (1996) Toward a theory regarding the pathogenesis of the systemic inflammatory response syndrome: what we do and do not know about cytokine regulation. Crit Care Med 24:163-172
9. Baue AE (1992) The horror autotoxicus and multiple organ failure. Arch Surg 127:1451-1462
10. Tompkins RG (1997) The role of proinflammatory cytokines in inflammatory and metabolic responses. Ann Surg 225(3):243-245
11. Roumen MH, Redl H, Schlag G et al (1995) Inflammatory mediators in relation to the development of multiple organ failure in patients after severe blunt trauma. Crit Care Med 23(3):474-480

12. Remick D, Manohar P, Bolgos G et al (1995) Blockade of tumor necrosis factor reduces lipopolysaccharide lethality, but not the lethality of cecal ligation and puncture. Shock 2(2):89-95
13. Riché F, Panis Y, Laisné M-J et al (1996) High tumor necrosis factor serum level is associated with increased survival in patients with abdominal septic shock: A prospective study in 59 patients. Surgery 120(5):801-807
14. Castelli MP, Black PL, Schneider M et al (1988) Protective, restorative, and therapeutic properties of recombinant human IL-1 in rodent models. J Immunol 140:3830
15. Cannon JG, Friedberg JS, Gelfand JA et al (1992) Circulating interleukin-1β and tumor necrosis factor-α concentrations after burn injury in humans. Crit Care Med 20(10): 1414-1419
16. O'Reilly M, Silver GM, Davis JH et al (1992) Interleukin 1β improves survival following cecal ligation and puncture. J Surg Res 52:518-522
17. Moscovitz H, Shofer F, Mignott H (1994) Plasma cytokine determinations in emergency department patients as a predictor of bacteremia and infectious disease severity. Crit Care Med 22(7):1102-1107
18. Kim JH, Jun TG, Sher TG (1995) Giant lymph node hyperplasia (Castelman's disease) in the chest. Ann Thorac Surg 59:1162-1165
19. Lange JR, Alexander HR, Merino MJ et al (1992) Interleukin-1 a prevention of the lethality of Escherichia Coli peritonitis. J Surg Res 52:555-559
20. León P, Redmond HP, Shou J et al (1992) Interleukin 1 and its relationship to endotoxin tolerance. Arch Surg 127:146-151
21. Luger A, Graf H, Schwarz H-P et al (1986) Decreased serum interleukin 1 activity and monocyte interleukin 1 production in patients with fatal sepsis. Crit Care Med 14(5):458-461
22. Echtenacher B, Männel DN, Hültner L (1996) Critical protective role of mast cells in a model of acute septic peritonitis. Nature 381:75-77
23. van der Poll T, Marchant A, Buurman WA et al (1995) Endogenous IL-10 protects mice from death during septic peritonitis. J Immunol 155:5397-5401
24. Greenberger MJ, Strieter RM, Kunkel SL et al (1995) Neutralization of IL-10 increases survival in a murine model of klebsiella pneumonia. J Immunol 155:722-729
25. Christou N, Meakins J, Gordon J et al (1995) The delayed hypersensitivity response and host resistance in surgical patients 20 years later. Ann Surg 222(4):534-548
26. Baue AE (1996) Prologue - The concept of limits and emergence of MOF. In: Faist E, Baue AE, Schildberg FW (eds) The immune consequences of trauma, shock and sepsis. Pabst Science Publishers, Berlin Germany, II-1:20-31

Sepsis and MODS - What Is Wrong and What Is Right

A. Gullo, G. Berlot

Despite major advances in the knowledge of the pathophysiologic mechanisms responsible of the develoment of sepsis and its related consequences, namely Multiple Organ Dysfunction Syndrome (MODS) and Failure (MOF), the mortality rate of septic patients remains high. Although this can be attributed to a number of factors, including the underlying diseases, a more advanced age of the affected patients, the appearance of antibiotic-resistant bacterial strains, etc., nevertheless it is surprising and somewhat disappointing that the clinical applications of the basic researches carried results far below the expectations [1]. Then, it appears rather logical to wonder a) if the measures developed to contrast sepsis, MODS and MOF on the basis of these experimental results are effective and b) if the main indicator used to assess the effectiveness of these approaches (namely the survival at a predetermined interval of time) is fully appropriate.

From the lab to the clinical arena

The gap existing between experimental findings and clinical results which are largely below the expectations is particularly evident when one takes in account the strategies developed against the mediators of sepsis.

The cardiorespiratory and metabolic derangements associated with the septic process are caused by the production and the release by the immunocompetent and the endothelial cells of a number of mediators deriving from the interaction between the infecting agent and the host [2, 3], including the tumour necrosis factor (TNF), the platelet activating factor (PAF), an ever-increasing number of interleukins (IL), the endothelin, the arachidonic acid derivates and many others. The same substances are also implicated in the development of the Systemic Inflammatory Response Syndrome (SIRS), when their activation is triggered by non-infectious events, including trauma, acute pancreatitis, ruptured aortic aneurysms, etc. [4]. However, not dissimilarly from other biological systems (e.g. the coagulative cascade), the secretion of many if not all of these mediators is counterbalanced by the contemporaneous release of inhibitory or blocking substances aimed to down-regulate the inflammatory process [5]. Basically, these agents acts by binding and inactivating the circulating septic mediators or by occupying their receptors on the surface of the target cells, thus making them unavailable for the active mediators [5]. To complicate further an already complex issue, it appears that in different stages of sepsis pro- and anti-inflammatory patterns of mediators can predominate, leading either to the the Mixed Antagonistic Response Syndrome (MARS) [6] or the Compensatory Anti Inflammatory Response Syndrome (CARS). This model can help to explain the reason(s) of the failure of the anti-mediators strategies proposed sofar. Actually, since the late '80s, the more in-depth knowledge of the basic pathophysiologic mechanisms underlying the septic process and the impressive progress of the genetic engineering techniques lead to the development of many substances able to blunt the effects of the septic mediators. This goal can be accomplished in different ways [7]. First, the circulating endotoxin and the septic mediators can be inactivated by specific antibodies. Second, the cell receptors can be selectively blocked by specific antagonists. Finally, the bloodborne mediators can be blocked by the linking with soluble receptors identical to those present on the cell surface. It is evident that, in many cases, these strategies reflect what is already occurring spontaneously in septic organisms. Despite the sound pathophysiologic basis and the promising experimental data, the overall results deriving from many large double blind, placebo-controlled clinical trials using different anti-mediators strategies have been sofar disappointing or far below the expectations, since some beneficial effects could be demonstrated only in certain subgroups of patients [1]. Moreover, some trials had to be suspended when an interim analysis demonstrated an excess mortality in the treatment group [1].

A number of anti-endotoxin antibodies were the first agents to be studied. At the beginning of the '80s Ziegler et al. [8], showed that an increased survival was associated with the administration of human polyclonal antibodies against the lipid A (J5). These results were confirmed by two other clinical studies which utilized polyclonal antiendotoxin antibodies derived form pooled sera [9, 10]. This approach had some limitations, including the instability of the solution, in the difficulty of measuring the real protective effect of a polyclonal preparation and in the risk of transmissible diseases [11]. The recent, impressive development of the genetic techniques allowed to overcome these inconveniences, and, ten years later, a better outcome was demonstrated in septic patients given monoclonal antiendotoxin antibodies enrolled in two large, multicenter, double blind, placebo-controlled studies. The first trial involved 486 patients with suspected Gram- sepsis who received E5, a murine monoclonal IgM anti lipid A antibody or placebo [12]. Even if the overall mortality rate was comparable in the two groups, in the subset of patients with confirmed Gram- septic shock mortality was slightly higher in the placebo group, whereas it was significantly lower in treated patients with sepsis but not in shock. In the same period, another trial was performed using a human monoclonal IgM antiendotoxin antibodies (HA-1A) (given as a single bolus of 100 mg i.v.) [13]. A subsequent analysis of data demonstrated that HA-1A was particularly effective in patients with higher blood endotoxin levels [11]. However, a confirmatory study with E5 failed to demonstrate any effect on survival, even if its administration was associated with a greater resolution of organ failure [14]. After publication of the study, some doubts had been raised about the results of the HA-1A study [15]. The areas of major concern were the randomization and the concomitant treatment (the placebo group was older, had a higher APACHE II score and had a higher rate of inadequate antibioticotherapy). In order to test its efficacy definitively, another multicenter, double blind study was started, using HA-1A. However, an interim analysis of data demonstrated a slight and nonsignificant excess of mortality in non-bacteremic patients given HA-1A, and the study was suspended [1].

Other clinical trials which involved anti-mediators agents shared the same destiny. Once again, the results expected on the basis of the laboratory findings were quite different from those observed clinically. Several investigations were addressed toward the possible therapeutic effects of the blockade of TNF in septic patients. Experimentally, antibodies directed against TNF exert a protective cardiovascular effects in animal models of septic shock [16]. Early clinical experiences were encouraging by indicating sometimes a rise in arterial pressure [17] and an improvement in left ventricular function [18]. A preliminary clinical trial involving only 42 patients was then performed, and the administration of anti-TNF antibodies was demonstrated to be free of harmful side effects and was associated with a substantial decrease of the circulating TNF molecules [19]. Unfortunately, two large, double-blind, placebo controlled trials with different anti-TNF antibodies failed to demonstrate any effect on the mortality of septic patients [20, 21]. However, in one of these studies, when treated patients were retrospectively divided in subgroups, an improved outcome could be demonstrated in patients with elevated baseline plasma levels of IL-6 [21]. A confirmatory trial was then launched, in which only septic patients with plasma IL-6 levels > 1000 pg/mL were enrolled. The study was suspended by the regulatory authorities when an interim analisis demonstrated that the results were inconclusive.

The inactivation of the septic mediators can be accomplished also by the administration of agents able to selectively block the receptors on the cell surface, making them unavailable for the active substance or by the interaction with specific circulating receptors, which bind the mediator, thus preventing the contact with the target cell. The IL-1ra has been also isolated in healthy volunteers given endotoxin [22]. So far, a number of trials using the receptor blocking agent of the IL-1 (IL-1ra), the soluble receptor of TNF and the PAF receptor antagonist have been performed. The potentially beneficial effects of this substance have been experimentally demonstrated in many experimental studies [23-26]. Then, on the basis of these encouraging results, some clinical trials of IL-1ra in septic patients have been implemented. A randomized, open-label multicenter Phase II study was performed in the US and involved 99 septic patients, who were given an initial loading dose of IL-1ra or placebo, followed by a 72-hour continuous infusion or one of three different doses (17, 67 or 133 mg/hr, respectively) or placebo [27]. The endpoint of the study was the survival at 28 days. In the treatment group, a dose-related increase of the survival was observed, being the mortality 44% in the placebo group, 32% in patients receiving the lowest dosage, 25% in patients receiving the intermediate dosage and 16% in patients receiving the highest dosage. At the end of the infusion, the severity of the disease, as expressed by the APACHE II score, was reduced in the treatment group. On the basis of these results, a larger, randomized, double blind, placebo controlled Phase III trial was launched. The trial involved 893 patients, who received either placebo or IL1-ra, which was administered as an intravenous loading dose of 100 mg followed by a 3-day infusion at two different dosages (1 or 2 mg/kg/hr, respectively) [28]. Unfortunately, the results of this study failed to confirm those of the previous one. Actually, no significant reduction of mortality was observed in the treated patients as compared with the controls (29% vs 35%, respectively). Some secondary and retrospective analyses demonstrated a better outcome in patients with dysfunction of one or more organs or in patients with a predicted risk of mortality $\geq 24\%$ [28, 29]. The results of these studies were so different that a second Phase III study was then performed, on the assumption that if the trend toward a better outcome could be demonstrated by a more sophisticated statistical analysis, then the IL1-ra could be clinically valuable, at least in selected subgroups of patients. However, a more recent confirmatory trial failed to demonstrate any beneficial effect of the IL1-ra in septic patients [30].

With the aim to contrast the systemic effects of TNF, other investigations were directed toward the effects of its soluble receptors. In septic organisms, the effects of TNF are mediated through 55-kd (TNFR I) and 75-kd (TNFR II) receptors, whose extracellular domain is shed from the cells during sepsis and, once released into the interstitial space and in the bloodstream, bind the circulating TNF molecules, thus preventing them to exert their effects [31]. Experimentally, the administration of soluble TNF receptors is associated with the attenuation of the increased pulmonary permeability and the neutrophil sequestration induced by an intestinal ischaemia-reperfusion injury [32]. However, as indicated by Van Zee et al. [33], the possible clinical utility of the soluble TNF receptors could be severely limited by their short half-life (minutes) and by the fact that the active TNF-α circulates as a trimeric molecule, and it is necessary to block at least two of its components to inactivate it. To overcome these shortcomings, recombinant TNF-α receptors have been linked to the FC and hinge regions of a human IgG molecule (TNFR:Fc) [34]. Two clinical trials tested the hypothesis that these fusion molecules could be useful in septic patients. In the first trial, the TNFR II:Fc was administered to patients with septic shock in three different dosages vs placebo [35]. Even if a dose-response relation between treatment and mortality was observed, no difference of mortality could be demonstrated between the control and the three treatment groups. Moreover, an excess mortality was observed in patients with Gram+ infections receiving the highest dosage. Another clinical trial was then performed, using the fusion molecule TNF I:Fc, again at three different dosages vs placebo [36]. The study involved 498 patients with severe sepsis and septic shock. The patients treated with the lowest dosage presented an excess mortality as compared with the other groups and this arm of the study had to be discontinued at an interim analysis. Overall, there was a non-significant trend toward a reduced 28-days mortality in all the treatment groups. However, a preplanned logistic regression analysis to assess the effects of treatment on the 28-days mortality by means of predicted mortality and plasma IL-6 levels demonstrated a significant improved survival in patients with severe sepsis who received TNF I:Fc at the highest dosage as compared with the placebo group. These inconcludent results can be at least partially explained by the findings of Goldie et al. [37] who measured circulating concentrations of sepsis mediators and their antagonists, including IL-1ra and both TNFR I and II. Initial serum values of soluble TNF receptors but not of IL-1ra were higher in nonsurvivors, and IL-1ra was markedly more elevated in patients who developed septic shock. Moreover, these investigators observed that cytokine antagonists were present in concentrations 30- to 100.000-fold greater than their corresponding mediators. Overall, these results indicate that a) in circumstances associated with a systemic inflammatory reaction, including sepsis, burns and the postoperative status, the naturally-occurring antagonists of the sepsis mediators are produced in huge amounts, whose entity largely exceeds that of the target molecules, and b), the measured values of these antagonists are higher in nonsurvivors or in patients who will develop severe complications including sepsis and MODS. As a consequence, it is questionable if, in clinical conditions, the supply of exogenous antagonists could provide any additional protective effect.

Other investigations involved the antagonism of the PAF, which is a low molecular weight phospholipid which is produced by macrophages under the influence of endotoxin [38]. Experimentally, the administration of PAF is associated with the haemodynamic and metabolic features of septic shock [39], including hypotension, tachycardia, the increase of the microvascular permeability, a negative inotropic effect and the margination and aggregation of leukocytes and platelets. A number of natural as well as synthetic PAF inhibitors have been so far identified and some of them underwent both experimental and clinical evaluation, which allowed to enlight the effects of PAF in various target tissues. In rats given endotoxin the appearance of patchy necrotic bowel lesions is associated with a TNF-induced increase in PAF secretion [40]; these lesions were prevented by the pretreatment with a specific PAF antagonist [41]. In healthy volunteers treated with a PAF antagonist 18 hours before the i.v. administration of endotoxin, a reduced cardiovascular, metabolic and hormonal response was observed, in the absence of significant changes of the serum level of the sepsis mediators [42]. Recently, a large randomized, multicenter placebo-controlled, double blind clinical trial has been performed using the PAF receptor antagonist BN 52021, which was administered at a dosage of 120 mg every 12 hours for 4 days

[43]. There was a nonsignificant improvement of the 28-days survival in treatment group rate as compared with placebo group. However, when subgroups of patients were analyzed separately, a significant reduction of mortality was observed in patients with Gram- infections, either shocked or not. Conversely, no differences in the outcome were demonstrated between the placebo and the treatment groups in the absence of a Gram- sepsis.

What is wrong? The reason(s) of a failure

From the above quoted studies, it appears that despite the sound biological basis, the clinical results deriving from different anti-mediators strategies are apparently disappointing or, at least, far below the expectations. Probably, several reasons can explain these findings, and the recent reappraisal of steroids in the treatment of sepsis underlines the opportunity of reconsidering apparently disappointing findings [44, 45].

Is it a matter of timeframe?

The time factor potentially limits the effectiveness of the administration of substances with anti-mediators properties, and the availability of an appropriate biological marker of the severity of sepsis could represent a major advance. Unfortunately, at the present time the more appropriate method to monitor the evolution of sepsis is far from having been elucidated, as most of the presently used indicators of the inflammatory response, such as body temperature, white cell count, erythrocyte sedimentation rate or reactive C-protein concentration are rather unspecific, and the measurement of sepsis mediators is not yet widely available or reliable enough. Actually, even if persistently elevated serum levels of mediators have been associated either with the development of the Multiple Organ Dysfunction Syndrome (MODS) and with an increased mortality [46, 47], nevertheless their measurement presents some limitations, including the variability of the cellular response, the cost of the lab process, and their fluctuating secretion [39]. Some studies demonstrated that the monitoring of some substances could be valuable for the biological monitoring of septic patients. Recent investigations demonstrated that elevated blood levels of IL-6, which is produced by various cells including monocytes, macrophages have been related to the severity of sepsis and the mortality thus making the serial determinations of this cytokine a potential useful tool [49-52]. Similar considerations apply for procalcitonin (PCT) which is produced by a non-thyroideal source under a stressful stimulus and whose levels have correlated either with the occurrence of infection and sepsis and with the severity of injury and hypovolaemia [53-55]. Despite the biologic relevance, it is important to recall that there are some evidences suggesting that the measurement of the serum level of a certain mediator provides only limited information on what is going at the tissue level. First, it should be reminded that circulating levels of cytokines represent only the tip of the iceberg, being the rest already bound to the receptors of the target cells where they exert their biological effects [56]. As a consequence, the administration of anti-TNFab on the basis of elevated circulating levels of this cytokine could be too late, as the biological effects as well as the interaction with other mediators have already occurred. Second, the pattern of mediators release and their biologic effects change with time. As stated above, it has been hypothesized that the clinical course of sepsis could be characterized by different stages of immunologic response, the MARS, in which inflammatory and anti-inflammatory substances are produced and released together, and the CARS, in which anti-inflammatory substances predominate, eventually leading to a down-regulation of the immunologic properties of the host. Then, one could take advantage from giving the appropriate mediator(s) or anti-mediator(s) according to the stage of the disease. As an example, in the MARS stage, the blockade of TNF or IL-1 could be effective as well as the administration of IL-10 or IL-11, which exert a powerful anti-inflammatory action [48]. Third, as the various sepsis mediators form a network characterized by many positive and negative feed-back loops, it is unlikely that the blockade of a single substance could give dramatic results. Then, not dissimilarly from the current treatment of neoplastic or infective diseases, future treatments could consist in cocktail of anti-mediators substances [48].

Is it a matter of analysis of the results?

Analyzing all published clinical studies involving anti-mediators agent, Zeni et al. [44] demonstrated that a) the mortality rate of the control groups is rather constant throughout the different trials, ranging from 35 to 40%, with the exception of an anti-PAF study, whose mortality peaked up to 50%; and b) in several cases there is a small, nonsignificant better survival in the treated patients (odds ratio 1.11; 95% interval of confidence (CI) 0.99 to 1.23; $p = 0.07$). However, by excluding the patients who received the highest doses of soluble TNF receptors and who showed the highest mortality, a small but significant improvement of survival appears (odds ratio 1. 12; CI 1.01 to 1.25; $p = 0.04$). Then, according to the authors, it could be possible that the enrollment of more patients (as many as 6-7000 for each trial) , and the use of lower doses of some agents (i.e. the TNF soluble receptor) could carry the long-expected encouraging results.

Is it a matter of design of the studies?

The 28-day outcome could have not been the most appropriate study endpoint. Actually, since sepsis is an extremely complex syndrome and survival is heavily influenced by factors other than the ongoing acute disorders, including age, pre-existing chronic diseases, etc., it is likely that in many cases the final outcome could be scarcely affected by this novel therapeutic approach. Actually, as recently demonstrated by Sprung et al. [57] by rewieving the database from a previous trial, as many as 22% of enrolled patients had their treatment withhold or withdrawn due to severity of their conditions, which made survival extremely unlike. More than 50% of these patients had severe underlying conditions carrying a poor prognosis, which probably could have vanished any effect on survival exerted by the anti-mediators strategy. Then, it is arguable that, had other markers of action been chosen, results could have been different. Actually, several experimental and clinical studies demonstrated that the same substances which turned out to be ineffective in modifying the outcome of septic patients can exert indeed some physiological desirable effects, as demonstrated either in rabbits in whom the administration of IL1-ra is able to reduce the derangement of the blood flow to vital organs occurring in experimental pancreatitis [58] and in septic patients, in whom the administration of an anti-TNF antibody can improve the cardiovascular function [18]. Similarly, it is possible that the administration of TNF-derived fusion protein could be effective in reducing the systemic inflammatory reaction of septic patients without influencing the final outcome, as recently demonstrated in patients with severe rheumatoid arthritis [59].

Conclusions

The administration of anti-mediators agents did not modify substantially the outcome of septic patients enrolled in several large controlled clinical trials. However, there are some evidences suggesting that these apparently disappointing results could have been different if more patients had been enrolled and/or endpoints different from survival had been chosen.

References

1. Bernard GR (1995) Sepsis trials. Am J Resp Crit Care Med 102:4-10
2. Rackow EC, Astiz ME (1991) Pathophysiology and treatment of septic shock. JAMA 266: 548-554
3. Berlot G, Vincent JL (1992) Cardiovascular effects of cytokines. Clin Intens Care 3:199-205
4. Davies MG, Hagen PO (1997) Systemic inflammatory response syndrome. Br J Surg 84: 920-935
5. Moldawer LL (1994) Biology of proinflammatory cytokines and their antagonist. Crit Care Med 22:S3-S7
6. Bone RC (1996) Sir Isaac Newton, Sepsis, SIRS and CARS. Crit Care Med 24:1125-1136
7. Christman JW, Holden EP, Blackwell TS (1995) Strategies for blocking the systemic effects of cytokines in the sepsis syndrome. Crit Care Med 23:955-963
8. Ziegler EJ, McCuchan JA, Fierer J et al (1982) Treatment of gram-bacteremia and shock with human antiserum to a mutant Escherichia coli. New Engl J Med 307:1225-1230
9. Lachman E, Pitsoe SB, Gaffin SL (1984) Antilypolisaccharide immunotherapy in the management of septic shock of obstetrical and gynecological origin. Lancet 1:981-983

10. Fomsgaard A, Baek L, Foomsgard JS et al (1988) Preliminary study in treatment of septic shock patients with antilypolisaccharide IgG with from blood donors. Scand J Infect Dis 21:697-708

11. Talan DA (1993) Recent developments in our understanding of sepsis: evaluation of antiendo-toxin antibodies and biological response modifiers. Ann Emer Med 22:1871-1990

12. Greenman RL, Schein RMH, Martin MA et al (1991) A controlled clinical trial of E5 murine monoclonal IgM antibody to endotoxin in the treatment of Gram- sepsis. JAMA 266:1097-1102

13. Ziegler EJ, McCutchan JA, Fierer J et al (1991) Treatment of Gram- bacteremia and septic shock with HA-1A human monoclonal antibody against endotoxin. A randomized, double blind, placebo controlled trial. N Engl J Med 324:429-436

14. Bone RC, Balk RA, Fein AM et al (1995) A second large controlled clinical study of E5, a monoclonal antibody to endotoxin: results of a prospective, multicenter, randomized, con-trolled study. Crit Care Med 23:994-1006

15. Cunnion RE (1992) Clinical trials of immunotherapy for sepsis. Crit Care Med 20:721-723

16. Silva AT, Bayston KF, Cohen J (1990) Prophylactic and therapeutic effects of a monoclonal antibody to tumour necrosis factor-alfa in experimental Gram- shock. J Inf Dis 162:421-427

17. Exley AR, Cohen J, Buurman WA et al (1990) Monoclonal antibody to TNF in severe septic shock. Lancet 335:1275-1277

18. Vincent JL, Bakker J, Marecaux G et al (1992) Administration of anti TNF antibodies im-proves left ventricular function in septic shock patients: results of a pilot study. Chest 101:810-815

19. Dhainaut JFA, Vincent JL, Richard C et al (1995) DP 571, a humanized antibody to tumour necrosis factor-alpha: safety, pharmacokinetics, immune response, and influence of the anti-body on cytokine concentrations in patients with septic shock. Crit Care Med 23:1461-1469

20. Cohen J, Carlet J for the INTERSEPT group (1996) INTERSEPT: an international, multicen-ter, placebo-controlled trial of monoclonal antibody to human tumor necrosis factor-α in pa-tients with sepsis. Crit Care Med 24:1431-1440

21. Rheinhart K, Wiegand-Lohnert C, Grimminger F et al (1996) Assessment of the safety and efficacy of the monoclonal anti-tumour necrosis factor antibody fragment, MAK 195F, in pa-tients with sepsis and septic shock: a multicenter, randomized, placebo-controlled, dose rang-ing study. Crit Care Med 24:733-742

22. Granowitz EV, Santos AA, Poutsaka DD et al (1991) Production of Interleukin-1 receptor an-tagonist during experimental endotoxemia. Lancet 1338:1423-1424

23. Dinarello CA (1991) The proinflammatory cytokines Interleukin-1 and Tumor Necrosis Fac-tor and treatment of septic shock syndrome. J Inf Dis 163:1177-1184

24. Ohlsson K, Bjork P, Bergenfeldt M et al (1990) Interleukin-1 receptor antagonist reduces mortality from endotoxin shock. Nature 343:550-552

25. Arend WP (1991): Interleukin 1 receptor antagonist: a new member of Interleukin 1 family. J Clin Invest 88:1445-1451

26. Fisher E, Marana MA, Van Zee KJ et al (1992) Interleukin-1 receptor antagonist improves survival and hemodynamic performance in Escherichia coli septic shock, but fails to alter host responses to sublethal endotoxemia. J Clin Invest 89:1551-1557

27. Fisher CJ, Slotman GJ, Opal SM et al (1994) Initial evaluation of human recombinant Inter-leukin 1 receptor antagonist in the treatment of sepsis syndrome: a randomized, open label, placebo-controlled multicentre trial. Crit Care Med 22:12-21

28. Fisher CJ, Dhainaut JF, Opal SM et al (1994) Recombinant human interleukin 1 receptor an-tagonist in the treatment of patients with sepsis syndrome. Results from a randomized, double blind, placebo-controlled trial. JAMA 271:1836-1843

29. Knaus WA, Harrell FE, LeBreque JF et al (1996) Use of predicted risk of mortality to evalu-ate the efficacy of anticytokine therapy in sepsis. Crit Care Med 24:46-56

30. Opal SM, Fisher CJ, Dhainaut JFA et al (1997) Confirmatory Interleukin-1 receptor antago-nist trial in severe sepsis: a phase III, randomized, double blind, placebo-controlled, multicen-ter trial. Crit Care Med 25:1115-1124

31. Bazzoni F, Beutler B (1996) Seminars in Medicine at the Beth Israel Hospital, Boston: The Tumour Necrosis factor ligand and receptor families. New Engl J Med 34:1717-1725
32. Sorkine P, Setton A, Halpern P et al (1995) Soluble tumour necrosis factor receptors reduce bowel ischemia-induced lung permeability and neutrophil sequestration. Crit Care Med 23: 1377-1381
33. Van Zee KJ, Kohno T, Fisher E et al (1992) Tumour necrosis factor soluble receptors circulate during experimental and clinical inflammation and can protect against excessive tumour necrosis factor alpha in vitro and in vivo. Proc Natl Acad Sci USA 89:4845-4849
34. Mohler KM, Torrance DS, Smith CA et al (1993) Soluble tumour necrosis factor (TNF) receptors are effective therapeutic agents in lethal endotoxemia and function simultaneously as both TNF carriers and TNF antagonists. J Immunol 151:1548-1561
35. Fisher CJ, Agosti JA, Opal SM et al (1996) Treatment of septic shock with the tumor necrosis factor receptor:Fc fusion protein. New Engl J Med 334:1697-1702
36. Abraham E, Glauser MP, Butler T et al (1997) p55 Tumor necrosis factor receptor fusion protein in the treatment of patients with severe sepsis and septic shock. A randomized controlled multicenter trial. JAMA 277:1531-1538
37. Goldie AS, Fearon KC, Ross JA et al (1995) Natural cytokine antagonists and endogenous antiendotoxin core antibodies in sepsis syndrome. JAMA 274:172-177
38. Bone RC (1992) Phospholipids and their inhibitors: a critical evaluation of their role in the treatment of sepsis. Crit Care Med 20:884-890
39. Lefer A (1989) Significance of lipid mediators in shock states. Circ Shock 27:3-12
40. Sun X, Hsueh W (1988) Bowel necrosis induced by tumour necrosis factor in rats is mediated by platelet activating factor. J Clin Invest 81:1328-1331
41. Sun X, Hsueh W, Torre-Amione G (1990) Effects of in vivo priming on endotoxin induced hypotension and tissue injury: the role of PAF and tumour necrosis factor. Am J Pathol 136: 949-956
42. Thompson WA, Coyle S, Van Zee K et al (1994) The metabolic effects of platelet activating factor in endotoxemic man. Arch Surg 129:72-79
43. Dhainaut JFA, Tenaillon A, Le Tulzo Y et al (1994) Platelet-activating factor antagonist BN 52021 in the treatment of severe sepsis: a randomized, double-blind, placebo-controlled, multicenter clinical trial. Crit Care Med 22:1720-1728
44. Zeni F, Freeman B, Natanson C (1997) Anti-inflammatory therapies to treat sepsis and septic shock: a reassessment. Crit Care Med 25:1095-1100
45. Bollaert PE, Charpentier C, Levy B et al (1998) Reversal of late septic shock with supraphysiologic doses of hydrocortisone. Crit Care Med 26:645-650
46. Pinsky MR, Vincent JL, Deviere J et al (1993) Serum cytokine levels in human septic shock: relation to multiple system organ failure and mortality. Chest 103:565-575
47. Calandra T, Baumgartner JD, Grau GE et al (1990) Prognostic values of tumour necrosis factor/cachectin, interleukin-1, interferon-alpha, and interferon gamma in the serum of patients with septic shock. J Infect Dis 161:982-987
48. Cain BS, Meldrum DR, Harken AH, McIntyre (1998) The physiologic basis for anticytokine clinical trials in the treatment of sepsis. J Am Coll Surg 186:337-350
49. Fassbender K, Pargger H, Muller W, Zimmerli W (1993) IL-6 and acute phase protein concentrations in surgical intensive care unit patients: diagnostic sign in nosocomial infection. Crit Care Med 21:1175-1180
50. Waage A, Aasen AO (1992) Different role of cytokine mediators in septic shock related to meningococcal disease and surgery. Immunology 127:221-230
51. Calandra T, Gerain J, Heumann D et al (1991) High circulating levels of interleukin-6 in patients with septic shock evolution during sepsis, prognostic value and interplay with other cytokines. Am J Med 91:23-29
52. Wakefield CH, Barclay GR, Fearon KCH et al (1998) Proinflammatory mediator activity, endogenous agonists and the systemic inflammatory response in intra-abdominal sepsis. Br J Surg 85:818-825

53. Dandona P, Nix D, Wilson MF et al (1994) Procalcitonin increase after endotoxin injection in normal subjects. J Clin Endocrinol Metab 79:1605-1608

54. Assicot M, Gendrel D, Carsin H et al (1993) High serum procalcitonin concentrations in patients with sepsis and infection. Lancet 341:515-518

55. Mimoz O, Benoist JF, Edouard AR et al (1998) Procalcitonin and C-reactive protein during the early postraumatic systemic inflammatory response syndrome. Intens Care Med 24: 185-188

56. Cavaillon JM, Munoz C, Fitting C et al (1992) Circulating cytokines: the tip of the iceberg? Circ Shock 38:145-152

57. Sprung CL, Eidelman LA, Pizov R et al (1997) Influence of alterations in forgoing life-sustaining treatment practices on clinical sepsis trial. Crit Care Med 25:383-387

58. Tanaka N, Murata A, Ken-ichi U et al (1995) Interleukin 1 receptor antagonist modifies the changes to vital organs induced by acute necrotizing pancreatitis in a rat experimental model. Crit Care Med 23:901-908

59. Moreland LA, Baumgartner SW, Schiff MH et al (1997) Treatment of rheumatoid arthritis with a recombinant human tumour necrosis factor receptor (p75)-Fc fusion protein. New Engl J Med 337:141-147

What Is Clinical Relevance? - Well Controlled Experiments in Normal Animals as Compared to Clinical Studies in Diverse Sick Patients

A.E. BAUE

> "KNOW then thyself,
> Presume not God to scan;
> The proper study of mankind is man".

Alexander Pope
An Essay on Man 1733-34 Epistle II.I

There has been recent emphasis on performing animal studies that are clinically relevant. It has been said that some of the clinical trials of so-called "magic bullets" may not have been carried out if appropriate or relevant trials had been carried out beforehand in animals. Evidence-based or critical appraisal animal research has also been described [1]. This is an incredible expression because – what is research if it isn't to provide evidence? It is now recommended also that we should practice evidence-based medicine [2].

Animal research has made an immense contribution to scientific knowledge and to the intricacies and development of, or solution to, biologic problems. Technical problems have been solved by study of such things as cardiopulmonary bypass and transplantation and an immense amount has been learned about shock, injury and inflammation. It has not been easy to translate this information in to better clinical care of patients. This is easy to understand. The complexities of human disease and patient care are difficult to deal with on a scientific research or protocol approach. Deitch has thoroughly reviewed and clearly identified the problems with clinical relevance of many, if not all, previous animal studies related to "magic bullets" [3]. He has clearly identified what is not clinically relevant. The question then is, what is clinically relevant? What are clinically relevant animal models? Is there such a thing? I have modified Table 8 in Deitch's publication (Table 1). It is an excellent comparison of the problems with animal and clinical research. I will emphasize several of these points.

Is there then any such thing as a clinically relevant animal study? Animal research is carried out in young, healthy animals. Why not use sick animals for a trial? How would you know then what helped and what did or did not kill the animals?

Table 1. Comparison of experimental models versus clinical realities

Experimental models	Clinical reality
Homogeneous genetic pool of a single sex	Heterogeneous genetic pool of two sexes
Species differences (mouse/rat/guinea pig/pig/dog)	Human studies
Pretreatment common (knock-out species is a variant of this strategy)	In patients, you cannot treat what is not there (or at least a great likelihood to be there soon)
Adjuvant therapy often not fully rendered: no resuscitation, no antibiotics, no organ support	Patients are always actively treated
Relevance of model to human disease:	Human disease:
a) Route of infection - i.v. versus natural	a) Patients are always infected through natural means - they are not deliberately infected
b) Use of avirulent versus virulent bacteria	b) Infecting bacteria are almost always virulent
c) Type of shock model (controlled versus uncontrolled haemorrhage, reversible versus irreversible)	c) Haemorrhagic shock is due to uncontrolled haemorrhage and we assume it is always reversible
d) Insult is uniform (all animals get the same dose of bacteria, LPS, etc.)	d) Patients' degrees of insult vary
e) Imposed temporal course of insultr	e) Disease follows a natural progression over an individualized time course
Endpoints may not represent clinical relevance (e.g., surrogate markers)	Clinically relevant endpoints are observable (i.e. improved organ function, improved mortality, etc.)
Study design may introduce clinically irrelevant variables (heparinization, anaesthesia, post hoc data analyses)	Patient care require optimal active care (i.e. do not heparinize haemorrhaging patients)
	Different diseases

From: Deitch EA (1998) Animal models of sepsis and shock. A review and lessons learned. Shock 9(1):1-11. With permission

So the first problem for a relevant animal model is that they are done in normal animals. Secondly, the animals must be cared for in a way that protects them from suffering. The principles of care of laboratory animals are important. This is not realistic and/or relevant for certain clinical problems. In animal research a pathophysiologic insult is induced which will cause problems for the animal in a matter of minutes or hours. Therapy or modification of the induced stress is begun before, at, or shortly after the insult. Is this relevant?

I have said that if I knew I was about to receive a bolus intravenous injection of endotoxin I would take a monoclonal anti-TNF antibody or an anti-endotoxin antibody beforehand because the evidence indicates that I would be protected. However, if I thought I was developing appendicitis or peritonitis, I would avoid such antibodies because the evidence suggests that they would increase mortality. Thus, too much may be bad but too little may be even worse. I have called these biologic conundrums or puzzles [4].

Another problem with animal models is that everyone wants to develop their own model. Some models have been used frequently such as our cecal ligation and puncture model in rats [5]. However, many other sepsis models have been used as well. Lerner Hinshaw tried to get a consensus on sepsis models and his attempt failed [6]. Uniform haemorrhagic shock models were never established except for the three general types – volume loss control, blood pressure control, or uncontrolled bleeding. Why was there no agreement or consensus on a model? Initially you may think that this is due to human ego's "my model" or everyone marches to their own drum. However, there is an even more important factor, I think, and that is that none of the models is truly clinical relevant. Thus, there is striving to try to develop a better one.

Bauhofer et al. with Lorenz in Marberg, have tried to "close the gap" between clinical trials and randomized animal studies by careful clinical management in animal studies which simulate the complexities of clinical interactions [7].

Animal studies of agents which are of historic interest only

"All people are animals but
Not all animals are people".
Deutschman's Disclaimer to Deitch's First Law of Research

History is a valuable teacher. There are many agents that were exciting in the animal laboratory but never made it into clinical use and did not survive clinical trials. Thus, the present problem with "magic bullets" is not new to older investigators. Most of the agents studied earlier were studied extensively by many of us (Table 2). There were exciting moments in the laboratory when we thought these agents had specific effects. I have reviewed these in detail [8].

Low molecular weight dextran was wonderful to prevent sludging of blood with shock. However, when it was given to patients, it was no better than Ringer's lactate and at times it accentuated or contributed to acute renal failure. Clinical dextran (average molecular weight of 65,000) has never been in common clinical use. Hypertonic saline/dextran is now making a comeback for resuscitation [9]. Whether it becomes established clinically remains to be seen. Dibenzyline (phenoxybenzamine) was very interesting in the laboratory and protected animals, particularly dogs, in end-stage shock. When it was given to patients under controlled circumstances there was a decrease in oxygenation and its use was a disaster. For a time it was used to prepare patients for resection of a pheochromocytoma. THAM (tris-hydroxymethylaminomethane) to correct intracellular acidosis sounded like an exciting agent, but it never proved of clinical benefit. There was a study of THAM reported at the most recent meeting of the Critical Care Society which again found no benefit – an example of reinventing

Table 2. Areas of potential therapy which are now of historic interest only

Agent	Effect
LMWD - low molecular weight dextran	Prevent sludging of blood
Clinical dextran	Provide oncotic pressure
DMSO - dimethyl sulfoxide	Various therapeutic effects - an antioxidant
Dibenzyline (phenoxybenzamine)	To decrease vasoconstriction in shock with excessive vasoconstriction
THAM (TRIS hydroxymethyl aminomethane)	Correction of intracellular acidosis
2,3 - diphosphoglycerate (2,3- DPG)	Increase oxygen unloading in the periphery of the circulation
Polarizing solutions (homeopathic doses of Mg, K, insulin, glucose, steroids)	Help cells function but no particular benefit
Steroids	Treatment of septic shock
White blood (excessive Ringer's lactate solution)	Try to increase capillary blood flow
Buffers	Treat extracellular acidosis

the wheel [10]. 2,3-DPG (diphosphoglycerate) was exciting initially but no one really needs it. Polarizing solutions were of no help. Steroids for septic shock are gone. Too much white blood (Ringer's lactate) is bad. Buffers, sodium bicarbonate and other agents for extracellular acidosis are not necessary if you improve the circulation. Thus, many of these agents which kept investigators busy and led to many National Institutes of Health grants for a number of years all fell to naught. Other agents now, so-called magic bullets, may fall to naught simply because they do not have the strength individually to produce major effects or benefits.

Other problems of relevance

Other dissimilarities of many human diseases and animal models are shown in Table 3.

The selection of animal species is another problem in relevance. There is great variability in the response, circulation or metabolism of animals of different species. This is illustrated in Table 4. Some investigators maintain that our close ancestor, the baboon, is the most relevant animal [12]. Others maintain that the pig is metabolically close to man. The present problems of obesity in society suggest that this is true. Small animals have many popular features such as many animals can be used quickly and economically. Thus, there may be no totally appropriate species. Much can be learned about the biological response

Table 3. Problems in relevance

Illness develops in awake humans, not anaesthetized animals	
Some human problems develop suddenly	Perforated duodenal ulcer
Some human problems develop slowly	Appendicitis
Some human problems may develop slow or fast	Perforated diverticulitis
	Pancreatitis
A single insult in an animal (shock + trauma)	But multiple organ injury in patients
3-day mortality in animals	28 days in patients
Pretreatment models in animals	Ridiculous for patients
No animal ICU except for the sheep model of MOF developed by Regel et al. [11]	
There are few if any truly relevant natural animal models of human disease	
Young healthy genetically inbred animals	Older patients with chronic disease of the heart, lungs, liver, kidneys, and others

to an insult in many of them. Animal research adds to our scientific knowledge base if not to patient care.

Table 4. Animal Species

The Phylogenetic Scale (High Up) - Primates - Baboons
The Metabolic Scale - Pigs
The Big Animal Scale - Dogs - Sheep
The Small Animal Scale - Economical - Controllable - Genetically and immunologically pure - Large numbers for statistical significance

Contributions of animals to solving the scourges of mankind

Many of the great diseases of mankind, particularly specific communicable diseases, have been solved with the help of animal studies. The two areas where this has been most evident are in immunology and virology. I will use quotations (and references may be historically accurate but their bibliographic citations leave much to be desired) from the book *Two Centuries of American Medicine* by Bordley and Harvey [13] and will cite exact, early references where they are available (Bordley and Harvey). These contributions of animal studies have been immense and I will be able to cite only a few. Many others will probably be known to the reader.

When there is a disease in animals that is similar to that in man then the contribution can be immense. An excellent example of this is the similarity between cowpox and smallpox.

In the 1790s the English physician Edward Jenner decided to put an old wives' tale to an experimental test [14]. The gossip among the local farmers was that dairy maids who developed the blebs of cow pox on their hands never contracted smallpox. Between 1796 and 1798 Jenner inoculated 23 people with material obtained from cow pox sores and then demonstrated that the inoculated individuals were immune to smallpox [11, 13]. In present day terms his experiments were not well controlled but his conclusions were correct: inoculation with cow pox renders an individual immune to smallpox.

Many decades later Pasteur coined the term "vaccination" for such procedures to honor Jenner's important discovery (the Latin vacca = cow).

In 1891 Pasteur succeeded in preventing anthrax by inoculations with an attenuated anthrax bacillus. In 1885 he employed the same principle and was able to prevent the development of rabies in men who had been bitten by rabid dogs. In 1882 a young Russian biologist, Elie Metchnikoff, implanted a rose thorn in a transparent starfish larvae and found that inflammatory cells surrounded the rose thorn. He developed the concept of what he termed phagocytosis (cells that eat) in a transparent water flea Daphnia in which phagocytic blood cells engulfed and removed a fungus to which the water flea was susceptible.

The diphtheria bacillus was discovered in 1883 by Edwin Klebs. In 1889 Roux and Yersin, at the Pasteur Institute, found that diphtheria bacilli, when grown in a culture medium, produced a toxin which, when injected into animals in very small doses, produced the characteristic features of diphtheria and death of the animal. Roux also found that injecting a small dose of the toxin to a large animal such as a horse and then injecting increasing amounts produced immunity in the animal and the animal could tolerate enormous doses of the toxin. Von Behren and Kitasato, at the Cox Institute, found that the serum of horses immunized against diphtheria toxin would protect other animals and the first child was treated in 1891 by this method. Horses became favorite production lines for antibody. Other animals have been used such as cattle, sheep, and even smaller animals such as rabbits. Success with diphtheria led to the development of a tetanus antitoxin.

The injection of rattlesnake venom into rabbits led to Ewing's explanation that venomized blood lost the power of resisting invasive infection. This led to the discovery of complement by Bordet and Ehrlich in 1899.

In 1901, in New York, Simon Flexner, during a spinal meningitis epidemic, cultured the meningococcus *in vitro* and then transmitted the disease to monkeys. He produced an anti-serum in horses which prevented or modified the disease in monkeys and then in people.

The contribution of animal studies to the triumph over poliomyelitis is a wonderful example. Carl Landsteiner in 1908 transferred poliomyelitis from a spinal cord victim to monkeys. In 1909 Flexner did the same and transferred polio from one monkey to another. Flexner also in 1910 produced active immunity in monkeys but it was unreliable. Then, in 1922, he produced a non-fatal form of experimental poliomyelitis. At that time poliomyelitis virus was propagated in mouse brain tissue. The immense contribution of Enders, Robins, and Weller of Harvard was that they grew cell cultures of the poliomyelitis virus in human intestinal cells and in other cells [15]. They recognized the virus in culture by a dye so that test animals were no longer necessary and they measured the neutralizing capability of anti-serum. Monkeys were then replaced by test tubes and this immense contribution led to the triumph over poliomyelitis and the Nobel Prize for these individuals.

The tuberculin reaction and other problems were worked out by Koch using guinea pigs. The problems of anaphylaxis were also worked out in guinea pigs.

The importance of the thymus, lymphocytes and other immune responses was also worked out initially in animal studies. Medawar of London [16] and Robert Good at the University of Minnesota [17] with other colleagues reported almost simultaneously on the results of removal of the thymus in newborn mice and rabbits. They found a reduction in the number of lymphocytes and the immunologic deficiency that this led to. Medawar also found that thymectomized animals could be returned toward normal by transplanting subcutaneously either syngeneic or allogeneic normal thymus tissue. The mice then did not reject the allogeneic graft and would accept subsequent tissue grafts from the same donor. Thus, modern immunology began. This shows the immense contribution of animal research to our understanding of the immune system.

Benacceraf at the NIH hooked a hapten onto poly-L-lysine and injected this into outbred guinea pigs. By these studies he demonstrated that responses were dependent on a single gene inherited as an autosomal dominant [18]. The contributions of animal studies to transplantation, to the immune response and other matters is well known to all. Immune complex disease was studied by Dixon and associates by passively transferring acute glomerulonephritis to monkeys by means of antibodies derived from human glomerular basement membranes.

Max Theiler confirmed the fact that yellow fever is caused by a filterable agent, a virus, and it could be transmitted to mice by intracerebral inoculation. The use of mice allowed a measurement of virus potency and also for measuring serum antibody levels by the virus-serum neutralization test developed by Sternberg. Immunity to a weakened yellow fever virus was developed in monkeys.

Salk's vaccine against poliomyelitis was thoroughly tested in animals [19]. The Salk vaccine had to be given by injection whereas the attenuated virus developed by Sabin could be given by mouth [20].

Fleming, in 1928, found that a mold had gotten into a culture and caused dissolution of staphylococci. He wrote a paper about it in 1929. The mold produced a substance that he called penicillin. This paper was forgotten until 1938 when Florey and Chain at Oxford found the paper, made some penicillin and found that it produced 100% survival in mice with virulent haemolytic streptococcus. The rest is history.

Other contributions have been made where the vector for a human disease has been found to be in animals or insects such as the Anopheles mosquito for malaria, rats and fleas, to people for plague, and other problems.

Summary: relevance

What then are the lessons from these experiences in terms of relevance? I conclude with the following:

1. If animals have the disease or are afflicted by the disease or have a similar disease, therapy can be studied in animals and that can be transposed to man.
2. If animals can be given the disease, or can transmit the disease, then therapy can be evaluated in those animals.
3. Animals or insects may serve as a reservoir for human disease.
4. Animals may be used to propagate an agent which causes a human disease.
5. Genetically inbred rats and mice are likely to be different from patients.

The commonality in all of these experiences is that these studies dealt with 1) specific diseases and 2) specific pathogens. Trying to reproduce in animals a clinical condition of man which is a more generalized process is difficult if not impossible. Gerd Regel developed a sheep model with multiple insults and a sheep intensive care unit in order to simulate the development of multiple organ failure after injury [11]. This is a difficult and expensive model and, although interesting, has so far not led to major contributions and solutions of the problem. It was a valiant effort, however.

If an animal is susceptible to a disease that also afflicts man such as with a bacteria, a virus or other agents and therapy works in the animal, then Koch's postulates can be fulfilled and it is a relevant model. However, in all of the scourges of mankind around the world, only smallpox has a very close animal similarity – cow pox. And, of course, from this Jenner developed a vaccine. Animals were important in poliomyelitis to grow the virus and to develop a vaccine. The Salk vaccine was a formalin killed virus grown in monkey kidneys. Malaria is transmitted by a mosquito and plague by fleas from rats. Tuberculosis also occurs in animals but therapy was not based on animal studies. Scurvy was solved in man. Penicillin is an antibiotic that showed possibilities *in vitro* and in animal studies. Digitalis (foxglove) was first used in patients. Thus, a final solution to a human disease may be suggested from animal studies. There may be ideas and possibilities, but the actual therapy eventually must be established in man.

Carefully controlled studies of various treatment modalities in normal animals with one perturbation, i.e. haemorrhage, cecal ligation and puncture (CLP), *E. coli* infusion and endotoxin infusion, or two perturbations, haemorrhage + fracture, burn + CLP, and therapy may yield statistically significant positive results but the results may be clinically irrelevant. The major reasons for this are variations in human disease such as the following: 1) the disease process – what is it? Pancreatitis is different from perforated diverticulitis and both differ from adult respiratory distress syndrome; 2) severity of disease; 3) extent of disease; 4) duration of disease; 5) remote organ function and chronic health problems; 6) age; 7) response of the individual; 8) complications; 9) therapy – timing, dose, duration; 10) other therapy or organ support.

Mark Clemens recently described the heterogeneity in biology which includes genetic diversity, differences in tissue, functional polarity and transmembrane gradients with maintenance of ion gradients. Finally, is there any such thing as a clinically relevant animal model? There are many animal models from which we gain important information. We can learn about many aspects of biology and the response of an organism. However, all we can get from animal models is suggestions, possibilities and directions. After thorough evaluation in a number of animals, we must begin then the search for relevance in patients or human volunteers by initial phase I studies of safety, phase II studies of safety in humans, and phase III studies in randomized trials in patients to see whether there is a difference or not. What should be the endpoints for such human trials is a matter for other and further discussions.

References

1. Piper RD, Cook DJ, Bone RC, Sibbald WJ (1996) Introducing critical appraisal to studies of animal models in investigating novel therapies in sepsis. Crit Care Med 24(12):2059-2070
2. Sackett DL, Rosenberg WMC (1995) The need for evidence-based medicine. J R Soc Med 88:620-624
3. Deitch EA (1998) Animal models of sepsis and shock. A review and lessons learned. Shock 9(1):1-11
4. Baue AE (1994) Organ dysfunction (MODS), organ failure (MOF) and therapeutic conundrums in injured and septic patients. In: A Gullo (ed) Sepsis and Organ Failure. Fogliazza, Milan 2:9-39
5. Wichterman KA, Baue AE, Chaudry IH (1980) Sepsis and septic shock - a review of laboratory models and a proposal. J Surg Res 29:189-201
6. Hinshaw L (1996) Mechanisms and therapy of endotoxin shock. Shock Tour Symposium Introductory Statement, Oklahoma State Med Assoc 59:407-484
7. Bauhofer A, Celik I, Gregor B et al (1977) Closing the gap between clinical trials and positive in vitro drug effects with randomized animal studies. Shock 5:47(A150)
8. Baue AE (1980) New concepts in shock therapy: Some clinical adventures and misadventures. In: AM Lefer, TM Saba, LM Mela (eds) Advances in Shock Research 3:67-76
9. Wade CE, Kramer GC, Grady JJ et al (1997) Efficacy of hypertonic 7.5% saline and 6% dextran 70 in treating trauma: a meta-analysis of controlled clinical studies. Surgery 122:609-616
10. Hin MH, Kupfer Y, Tessler S (1997) Hemodynamic effects of tromethamine in the treatment of severe metabolic acidosis. Crit Care Med 25:A105(228)
11. Grotz M, Regel G, Dwenger A et al (1995) A standardized large animal model of multiple organ failure after severe trauma. Unfallchirurg 98:63-71
12. Redl H, Schlag G, Bahraim S et al (1996) Animal models as the basis of pharmacologic intervention in trauma and sepsis patients. World J Surg 20:487-492

13. Bordley J III, Harvey AM (1976) Two Centuries of American Medicine 1776-1996. W.B. Saunders, Philadelphia
14. Jenner E (1976) Letter to CH Parry, M.D., June 21, 1798. In: Bordley J III, Harvey AM. Two Centuries of American Medicine 1776-1996. W.B. Saunders, Philadelphia
15. Enders JF, Weller TH, Robbins FC (1949) Cultivation of the Lansing strain of poliomyelitis virus in cultures of various human embryonic tissues. Science 109:85
16. Medawar PB (1974) The new immunology. Hosp Prac 9:48
17. Good RA, Finstod J (1967) The development and involution of the lymphoid system and immunologic capacity. Trans Am Clin Climatol Assoc 79:69
18. McDevitt HO, Benacceraf B (1969) Genetic control of specific immune responses. Adv Immunol 11:31
19. Salk JE (1955) Vaccines for poliomyelitis. Sci Am 192:42
20. Marks G, Beatty WK (1973) The Story of Medicine in America. Charles Scribner's Sons, New York

THE MARKERS OF SEPSIS

Apoptosis (Programmed Cell Death) and the Resolution of Acute Inflammation

A.H. Rouzati, R. Taneja, J.C. Marshall

Biology, for the clinician, has classically encompassed the study of the life and growth of cells and organisms; death has been perceived as a pathologic process to be prevented. But over the past few years, our perception of cell death has undergone a major transformation [1]. It is now recognized that cells do not have an absolute and unchangeable lifespan, but rather that cell survival can change in response to environmental stimuli. Moreover, a moment's reflection will confirm that for a host of normal biologic processes, controlled cellular death is not only inevitable, but critical to normal development. During embryogenesis, the formation of mature organs is dependent on the controlled remodeling of tissues resulting, for example, in the formation of interdigital web spaces or the canalization of the gastrointestinal tract. Deletion of autoreactive T cells during immune maturation is essential to prevent autoimmune disease; other tissues such as blood cells, and epithelial cells of the skin, or gastrointestinal tract are constantly formed and shed during life. The programmed death of cells is called *apoptosis*.

Apoptosis and necrosis

Cells can die a pathological or physiological death [2]. *Necrosis* is the pathological form of cell death, and not the mechanism by which cells usually die. Necrosis typically occurs when the environment of the cell is unable to support cellular metabolic needs, either because of an acute deficiency of a vital substrate such as oxygen or nutrients, or because of exposure to substances that are toxic to the vital processes of the cell. Necrosis is characterized by uncontrolled changes in cellular architecture and function, leading to the release of intracellular contents into the cellular microenvironment. The necrotic cell swells, and the membrane ruptures; intracellular contents evoke an inflammatory response, leading to the phagocytosis of cellular debris.

Apoptosis, on the other hand, is a tightly controlled process, initiated through the expression of an endogenous cell death program, and brought about through the sequential and co-ordinated action of intracellular enzymes. In contrast to the necrotic cell, the apoptotic cell shrinks, its chromatin condenses, and the intracellular contents become organized into membrane-bound organelles known as apoptotic bodies. These apoptotic bodies are rapidly and efficiently removed by cells of the reticuloendothelial system, without evoking an inflammatory response. The process of apoptosis proceeds rapidly in vivo, and may be missed in tissue sections, although apoptotic cells are recognized occasionally as pyknotic cells.

Mechanisms of apoptosis

Apoptosis is a highly conserved process in evolution. In fact, contemporary understanding of the cellular mechanisms of apoptosis is grounded in studies of the mechanisms of embryologic cell death in the nematode, *Caenorhabditis elegans*. During its maturation to an adult worm, *C. elegans* loses exactly 131 cells through apoptosis, leaving 959 cells [3] 2 genes, *ced-3* and *ced-4*, which stimulated apoptosis [4] and one gene, *ced-9*, which inhibited it [5]. A human homolog of *ced-9* was identified in a B-cell lymphoma and thus called bcl-2 [6]. Bcl-2 proved to be a mitochondrial protein involved in cytochrome c and calcium transport that served as an inhibitor of apoptosis in human cells [7]. It is now recognized as one of a larger family of proteins which includes proteins that both stimulate (*bax*) and inhibit (*bcl-2, bad*) apoptosis.

The search for a human *ced-3* homolog identified the interleukin-1β converting enzyme (ICE) as the first member of a family of intracellular proteins that are capable of inducing apoptosis [8]. To date, at least 11 members of this family have been identified [9]. All are cysteine proteases that share the common feature of cleaving their substrates at sites adjacent to aspartic acid residues. Proteins of this family have been termed *caspases* (cysteine proteases with aspartic acid targets) [10]; ICE is now more commonly referred to as caspase-1. Caspase targets within the cell include proteins ranging from DNA repair enzymes such as poly-ADP ribose polymerase to cytoskeletal proteins including actin; they also cleave pro-forms of each other, yielding active caspase enzymes.

Apoptosis proceeds spontaneously in a variety of cell types; the apoptotic program can also be induced through signals from the environment. For instance, the engagement of a cell surface receptor called Fas by its ligand, Fas ligand, leads to caspase activation and apoptosis [11]. Interactions between Fas and Fas ligand are responsible for the maintenance of immune privilege in anatomic environments such as the anterior chamber of the eye [12]. Conversely, deficiency of Fas or Fas ligand in animals [13] or humans [14] results in the development of autoimmunity. Another well known member of this family of cell surface death receptors is the receptor for the cytokine, tumour necrosis factor (TNF), whose engagement can also induce apoptosis [15, 16]. Indeed induction of apoptosis by TNF represents the mechanism of its anti-tumour activity [17].

The final consequence of initiation of the apoptotic program is nuclear fragmentation and plasma membrane changes leading to the formation of apoptotic bodies. The nuclear changes of apoptosis can be recognized through the formation of a characteristic ladder pattern on DNA gel electrophoresis, or by flow cytometry as reduced uptake of the nuclear dye, propidium iodide. Membrane changes of apoptosis include exteriorization of phosphatidyl serine, normally located on the inner aspect of the plasma membrane, detectable as binding of annexin V by flow cytometry [18].

Apoptosis in the pathogenesis of critical illness

Alterations in the expression of apoptosis – both acceleration and inhibition of the apoptotic program – appear to play a role in the pathogenesis of critical illness.

In 1995, Teodorczyk-Injeyan et al. showed that lymphocyte apoptosis is accelerated following burn injury, and is responsible for burn-associated lymphopenia [19]. Similar conclusions have been drawn in a rat model of burn injury in which enhanced thymocyte apoptosis is associated with immune dysfunction [20]. Fas-mediated apoptosis of circulating lymphocytes is also increased following major surgery [21].

Hepatocytes express the Fas receptor and are very sensitive to its stimulation [22]. As a result, various forms of liver injury have been associated with abnormalities in apoptosis. Apoptosis is thought to play an important role in such pathological conditions as toxic and metabolic liver injury (for example, alcoholic cirrhosis), immune-mediated injury (for example, host-versus-allograft reaction in allograft rejection) and various viral liver diseases [23]. Liver failure in patients suffering from viral fulminant hepatitis has been shown to be a result of the apoptotic death of Fas expressing hepatocytes [24]. Similarly, interactions between Fas and its physiologic ligand have been implicated in the pathogenesis of acute Wilson's disease, with activation of Fas as consequence of the interaction of the hepatocyte with copper [25]. Injection of mice with anti-Fas antibody results in fulminant liver failure as a consequence of increased hepatocyte apoptosis [26]. Furthermore, accelerated apoptosis has been implicated as the mechanism of tissue injury in the liver and spleen in experimental endotoxin shock [27].

Under normal physiologic conditions, the expression of apoptosis in the adult kidney is uncommon. However, apoptosis appears to play a role in a number of pathologic states. Experimental models of partial ureteric obstruction and renal artery stenosis reveal an important relationship between restricted renal blood supply and loss of renal mass due to apoptotic cell death [28]. Diabetes and hypertension associated renal damage have also been shown to involve apoptosis, as has immune mediated glomerulonephritis [29].

The exotoxin of *Clostridium difficile*, the causative agent of pseudomembranous colitis, has been demonstrated to induce the apoptosis of intestinal epithelial cells [30]. Inhibition of apoptosis by viral proteins is a common mechanism in acute viral infections [31, 32]. In contrast, HIV infection induces lymphopenia, in part, through the effects of the virus in upregulating expression of Fas ligand on host macrophages [33].

Delayed neutrophil apoptosis in systemic inflammation

Impaired expression of apoptosis may also contribute to the pathogenesis of critical illness. The development of a syndrome of sustained and exaggerated inflammation, popularly known as the Systemic Inflammatory Response Syndrome (SIRS) [34], is the predominant risk factor for the development of the multiple organ dysfunction syndrome (MODS), the leading cause of death in critical illness [35]. While infection is an important cause of SIRS, the syndrome can also develop following multiple trauma, burns, acute pancreatitis, major surgery, and other acute insults associated with the activation of an endogenous inflammatory response.

Through the release of proteases and toxic oxygen metabolites, neutrophils play an important role in the pathophysiology of SIRS as mediators of tissue injury and organ dysfunction [36, 37]. The lifespan of the neutrophil in vivo is short, probably not longer than 5 or 6 hours, and is terminated through the activation of a constitutively expressed cell death program that induces neutrophil apoptosis, and their removal by cells of the reticuloendothelial system [18]. Thus neutrophil-mediated inflammation is terminated through the programmed cell death of the neutrophil. Expression of apoptosis can be inhibited by a large number of inflammatory mediators of both microbial and host origin [38, 39]. The stimuli that inhibit the constitutive expression of neutrophil apoptosis are many, and include microbial products such as endotoxin and fMLP, cytokines such as IL-1β, IL-8, and GM-CSF, and the process of transmigration into an inflammatory focus, or the cross-linking of cell surface β2 integrins [40].

Neutrophil apoptosis and the pathogenesis of ARDS

Although the acute respiratory distress syndrome has been described in neutropenic patients [41], a large body of clinical and experimental data supports the concept that neutrophils contribute to the evolution of acute lung injury [42]. Autopsy studies typically show massive accumulation of neutrophils in the lungs of patients with ARDS, and, at least in ARDS associated with sepsis, non-survivors show persistently higher numbers of neutrophils on bronchoalveolar lavage [43]. Concentrations of the PMN chemoattractant, IL-8, are increased in BAL fluid, and correlate with both neutrophil counts and increased risk of mortality [44]. Neutrophils recovered from the lung of the patient with ARDS are activated, as manifested by increased expression of β2 integrins and shedding of L-selectin [45]. Moreover patients with ARDS have elevated levels of hydrogen peroxide in the exhaled gas [46]. Finally, there are at least two case reports documenting deterioration of ARDS in critically ill patients given G-CSF [47] or GM-CSF [48], cytokines that increase circulating neutrophil numbers by augmenting their release from the bone marrow, and by inhibiting apoptosis.

There is no evidence that neutrophils that have migrated into the injured lung are able to return to the blood stream, nor that lymphatic drainage provides an important disposal route [49]. Thus the removal of neutrophils from the lung in ARDS appears to require the apoptotic death of the cell [50]. Lung neutrophil apoptosis is delayed during experimental acute lung injury [51], as well as in patients with ARDS [52]. BAL fluid from patients with ARDS inhibits the apoptosis of control neutrophils, an effect that can be reversed with antibodies to G-CSF or GM-CSF [52]. Serial studies in ARDS have suggested that patients who survive ARDS following sepsis have an increase in alveolar macrophage neutrophil ratio over time [53], consistent with the removal of neutrophils by macrophages. The cytokine, IL-10, has also been shown to hasten the resolution of pulmonary inflammation by promoting the restoration of normal neutrophil apoptosis [54].

Neutrophil apoptosis in SIRS

Neutrophils collected from patients following burn injury showed delayed apoptosis; the apoptotic delay can be reversed with a neutralizing antibody to GM-CSF [55]. Similar observations have been made in victims of multiple trauma: delayed neutrophil apoptosis is partially reversed by neutralization of G-CSF, but not of GM-CSF [56]. Our group has shown that patients with SIRS, and patients who have undergone major elective surgery (elective repair of an abdominal aortic aneurysm), show delayed neutrophil apoptosis (Fig. 1), in association with evidence of neutrophil activation, reflected in augmented respiratory burst activity [57] (Fig. 2). This delay is at least partially mediated by antiapoptotic factors in the plasma, as plasma from patients with SIRS is able to delay the apoptosis of normal control neutrophils.

Conclusions

A better understanding of the mechanisms of apoptosis should lead to new approaches to treat a broad spectrum of diseases. New therapeutic strategies will emerge as the molecular mechanisms involved in the cell's program of apoptosis are defined. For example, caspase inhibitors have been shown to have a protective effect in animal models of apoptosis induced liver disease caused by en-

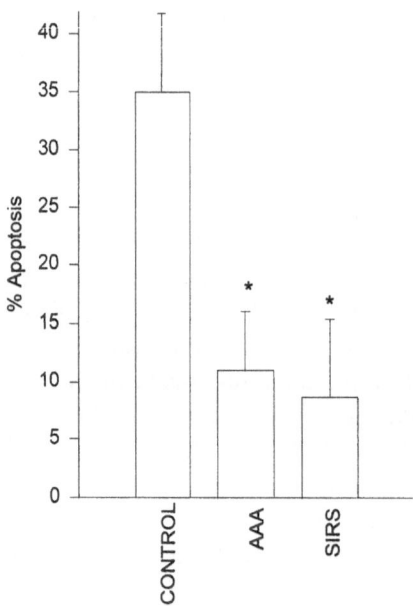

Fig. 1.
Expression of apoptosis is inhibited in patients with SIRS, or those who have undergone an elective repair of an abdominal aortic aneurysm. Rates of apoptosis were determined as the uptake of propidium iodide by flow cytometry. Modified from [57]

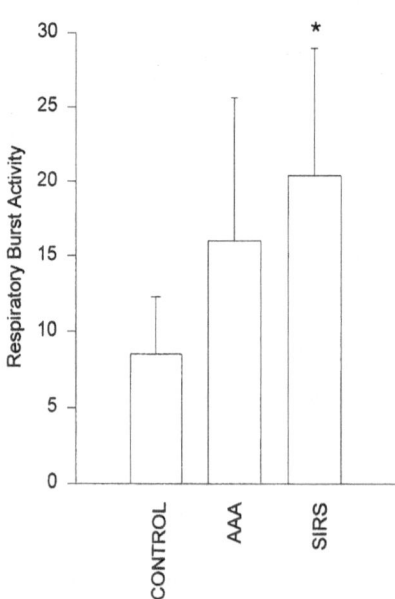

Fig. 2.
Concomitant with delayed apoptosis, neutrophils from patients with SIRS, or patients having undergone elective aneurysmectomy, show enhanced respiratory burst activity; data reflect log mean channel fluorescence of dihydrorhodamine 123. Modified from [57]

gagement of the Fas or TNF [58]. Other agents capable of modulating the expression of apoptosis may find a role in the treatment of SIRS in the ICU setting. For example, the normal expression of apoptosis in inflammatory neutrophils can be restored by inhibition of ICE [59], by IL-10 [54], or by inhibition of calpain [60]. Ironically, an improved understanding of the mechanisms of cell death may provide new insights into preventing mortality in the ICU.

References

1. Hetts SE (1998) To die or not to die: an overview of apoptosis and its role in disease. JAMA 279:300-307
2. Majno G, Joris I (1995) Apoptosis, oncosis, and necrosis. An overview of cell death. Am J Pathol 146:3-15
3. Ellis RE, Yuan J, Horvitz HR (1991) Mechanisms and function of cell death. Ann Rev Cell Dev Biol 7:663-698
4. Yuan J, Horvitz HR (1990) The Caenorhabditis elegans genes ced-3 and ced-4 act cell autonomously to cause programmed cell death. Dev Biol 138:33-41
5. Hengartner MO, Ellis RE, Horvitz HR (1992) Caenorhabditis elegans gene ced-9 protects cells from programmed cell death. Nature 356:494-499
6. Yang E, Korsmeyer SJ (1996) Molecular thanatopsis: A discourse on the Bcl-2 family and cell death. Blood 88:386-401
7. Yang J, Liu XS, Bhalla K et al (1997) Prevention of apoptosis by Bcl-2: Release of cytochrome c from mitochondria blocked. Science 275:1129-1132
8. Yuan J, Shaham S, Ledoux S et al (1993) The C. elegans cell death gene ced-3 encodes a protein similar to mammalian interleukin 1b converting enzyme. Cell 75:641-652
9. Alnemri ES (1997) Mammalian cell death proteases: a family of highly conserved aspartate specific cysteine proteases. J Cell Biochem 64:33-42
10. Alnemri ES, Livingston DJ, Nicholson DW et al (1996) Human ICE/CED-3 protease nomenclature. Cell 87:171
11. Nagata S, Golstein P (1995) The Fas death factor. Science 267:1449-1456
12. Griffith TS, Brunner T, Fletcher SM et al (1995) Fas ligand-induced apoptosis as a mechanism of immune privilege. Science 270:1189-1192
13. Takahashi T, Tanaka M, Brannan CI et al (1994) Generalized lymphoproliferative disease in mice, caused by a point mutation in the Fas ligand. Cell 76:969-976
14. Rieux-Laucat F, Le Deist F, Hivroz C et al (1995) Mutations in Fas associated with human lymphoproliferative syndrome and autoimmunity. Science 268:1347-1349
15. Boldin MP, Goncharov TM, Goltsev YV et al (1996) Involvement of MACH, a novel MORT1/FADD-interacting protease, in Fas/APO-1- and TNF receptor-induced cell death. Cell 85:803-815
16. Wallach D, Boldin M, Varfolomeev E et al (1997) Cell death induction by receptors of the TNF family: towards a molecular understanding. FEBS Lett 410:96-106
17. Woods KM, Chapes SK (1993) Three distinct cell phenotypes of induced-TNF cytotoxicity and their relationship to apoptosis. J Leuk Biol 53:37-44
18. Savill JS, Wyllie AH, Henson JE et al (1989) Macrophage phagocytosis of aging neutrophils in inflammation. J Clin Invest 83:865-875
19. Teodorczyk-Injeyan JA, Cembrznska-Nowak M, Lalani S et al (1995). Immune deficiency following thermal trauma is associated with apoptotic cell death. J Clin Immunol 15:318-328
20. Nakanishi T, Nishi Y, Sato EF et al (1998) Thermal injury induces thymocyte apoptosis in rats. J Trauma 44:143-148

21. Oka M, Hirazawa K, Yamamoto K et al (1996) Induction of Fas-mediated apoptosis on circulating lymphocytes by surgical stress. Ann Surg 223:434-440
22. Feldman G (1997) Liver apoptosis. J Hepatol 26:1-11
23. Galle PR (1997) Apoptosis in liver disease. J Hepatol 27:405-412
24. Galle PR, Hofmann WJ, Walczak H et al (1995) Involvement of the CD95(APO-1/Fas) receptor and ligand in liver damage. J Exp Med 182:1223-1230
25. Strand S, Hofmann WJ, Grambihler A et al (1998) Hepatic failure and liver cell damage in acute Wilson's disease involve CD95 (APO-1/Fas) mediated apoptosis. Nature Med 4:588-593
26. Lacronique V, Mignon A, Fabre M et al (1996) Bcl-2 protects against lethal hepatic apoptosis induced by an anti-Fas antibody in mice. Nature Med 2:80-86
27. Haendeler J, Messmer UK, Brune B et al (1996) Endotoxin shock leads to apoptosis in vivo and reduces bcl-2. Shock 6:405-409
28. Gobe GC, Axelsen RA, Searle JW (1990) Cellular events in experimental unilateral ischemic renal atrophy and in regeneration after contralateral nephrectomy. Lab Invest 56:770-779
29. Buttyan R, Gobe G (1997) Apoptosis in the mammalian kidney: incidence, effectors, and molecular control in normal developmental and disease states. Adv Pharmacol 41:369-381
30. Mahida YR, Makh S, Hyde S et al (1996) Effect of *Clostridium difficile* toxin A on human intestinal epithelial cells: induction of interleukin 8 production and apoptosis after cell detachment. Gut 38:337-347
31. Ray CA, Black RA, Kronheim SR et al (1992) Viral inhibition of inflammation: Cowpox virus encodes an inhibitor of the interleukin-1 beta converting enzyme. Cell 69:597-604
32. Leopardi R, Roizman B (1996) The herpes simplex virus major regulatory protein ICP4 blocks apoptosis induced by the virus or by hyperthermia. Cell Biol 93:9583-9587
33. Badley AD, McElhinny JA, Leibson PJ et al (1996) Upregulation of Fas ligand expression by human immunodeficiency virus in human macrophages mediates apoptosis of uninfected T lymphocytes. J Virol 70:199-206
34. Bone RC, Balk RA, Cerra FB et al (1992) Definitions for sepsis and organ failure and guidelines for the use of innovative therapies in sepsis. Chest 101:1644-1655
35. Beal AL, Cerra FB (1994) Multiple organ failure syndrome in the 1990's. Systemic inflammatory response and organ dysfunction. JAMA 271:226-233
36. Weiss SJ (1989) Tissue destruction by neutrophils. N Engl J Med 320:365-376
37. Fujishima S, Aikawa N (1995) Neutrophil-mediated tissue injury and its modulation. Intensive Care Med 21:277-285
38. Lee A, Whyte MKB, Haslett C et al (1993) Inhibition of apoptosis and prolongation of neutrophil functional longevity by inflammatory mediators. J Leuk Biol 54:283-288
39. Marshall JC, Watson RWG (1997) Programmed cell death (apoptosis) and the resolution of systemic inflammation. Can J Surg 40:169-174
40. Watson RWG, Rotstein OD, Nathens AB et al (1997) Neutrophil apoptosis is modulated by endothelial transmigration and adhesion molecule engagement. J Immunol 158:945-953
41. Ognibene FP, Martin SE, Parker MM (1986) Adult respiratory distress syndrome in patients with severe neutropenia. N Engl J Med 315:547-551
42. Windsor ACJ, Mullen PG, Fowler AA et al (1993) Role of the neutrophil in adult respiratory distress syndrome. Br J Surg 80:10-17
43. Steinberg KP, Milberg JA, Martin TR et al (1994) Evolution of bronchoalveolar cell populations in the adult respiratory distress syndrome. Am J Respir Crit Care Med 150:113-122
44. Miller EJ, Cohen AB, Nagao S et al (1992) Elevated levels of NAP-1/interleukin-8 are present in the airspaces of patients with the adult respiratory distress syndrome and are associated with increased mortality. Am Rev Respir Dis 146:427-432
45. Chollet-Martin S, Jourdain B, Gibert C et al (1996) Interactions between neutrophils and cytokines in blood and alveolar spaces during ARDS. Am J Respir Crit Care Med 154:594-601
46. Baldwin SR, Grum CM, Boxer LA et al (1986) Oxidant activity in expired breath of patients with adult respiratory distress syndrome. Lancet 1:11-14

47. Schilero GJ, Oropello J, Benjamin E (1995) Impairment in gas exchange after granulocyte colony stimulating factor (G-CSF) in a patient with the adult respiratory distress syndrome. Chest 107:276-278
48. Verhoef G, Boogaerts M (1991) Treatment with granulocyte-macrophage colony-stimulating factor and the adult respiratory distress syndrome. Am J Hematol 36:285-287
49. Weiland JE (1986) Lung neutrophils in adult respiratory distress syndrome. Clinical and pathologic significance. Am Rev Respir Dis 133:218-225
50. Cox GJ, Crossley J, Xing Z et al (1995) Macrophage engulfment of apoptotic neutrophils contributes to the resolution of acute pulmonary inflammation in vivo. Am J Respir Cell Mol Biol 12:232-237
51. Watson RWG, Rotstein OD, Parodo J et al (1997) Impaired apoptotic death signaling in inflammatory lung neutrophils is associated with decreased expression of interleukin 1b converting enzyme family proteases (caspases). Surgery 122:163-172
52. Matute-Bello G, Liles WC (1997) Neutrophil apoptosis in acute respiratory distress syndrome. Am J Respir Crit Care Med 156:1969-1977
53. Steinberg KP, Milberg JA, Martin TR et al (1994) Evolution of bronchoalveolar cell populations in the adult respiratory distress syndrome. Am J Respir Crit Care Med 150:113-122
54. Cox G (1996) IL-10 enchances resolution of pulmonary inflammation in vivo by promoting apoptosis of neutrophils. Am J Physiol 271: L566-L571
55. Chitnis D, Dickerson C, Munster AM et al (1996) Inhibition of apoptosis in polymorphonuclear neutrophils from burn patients. J Leuk Biol 59:835-839
56. Ertel W, Keel M, Infanger M et al (1998) Circulating mediators in serum of injured patients with septic complications inhibit neutrophil apoptosis through up-regulation of protein tyrosine phosphorylation. J Trauma 44:767-776
57. Jimenez MF, Watson RWG, Parodo J et al (1997) Dysregulated expression of neutrophil apoptosis in the systemic inflammatory response syndrome (SIRS). Arch Surg 132:1263-1270
58. Rouquet N, Pages JC, Molina T et al (1996) ICE inhibitor YVAD-cmk is a potent therapeutic agent against in vivo liver apoptosis. Curr Biol 6:1192-1195
59. Watson RWG, Rotstein OD, Parodo J et al (1998) The interleukin-1 beta converting enzyme (caspase-1) inhibits neutrophil apoptosis through processing of interleukin-1. J Immunol
60. Lu Q, Mellgren RL (1996) Calpain inhibitors and serine protease inhibitors can produce apoptosis in HL-60 cells. Arch Biochem Biophys 334:175-181

"Untimely Apoptosis" Is the Password

T.G. BUCHMAN

Multiple organ failure (also known as the multiple organ dysfunction syndrome [MODS]) remains a formidable foe. Despite advances in critical care including scoring systems, predictive models, monitoring, imaging and specific interventions, the mortality of multiple organ failure remains paradoxically high. The purpose of this brief chapter is to review what is known and consider what might be determined regarding apoptosis in MODS.

Apoptosis

Apoptosis [1] is a regulated process culminating in cell death which is essential to development, growth and maintenance of multicellular organisms. The purpose of apoptosis appears to be the efficient recycling of senescent and otherwise surplus cells while bypassing defensive programs such as inflammation. The process, and the network of genes regulating the process, have been conserved through evolution in part because they are essential to development: for example, the nematode *C. elegans* destroys more than 10% of its cells during its three day maturation. In humans, developmental apoptosis is responsible for such diverse processes as remodeling of the genitourinary tract and lysis of the interdigital webs. In the mature human, apoptosis is responsible for such critical maintenance functions as sloughing of intestinal epithelium at the villus tip, removal of surplus leukocytes and lymphocytes, and exfoliation of sun-damaged skin.

Errors in apoptosis can be roughly divided into two groups: errors in which apoptosis is delayed and errors in which apoptosis is triggered too early. Delayed apoptosis has been linked to human malignancies including colon cancer and B-cell-lymphoma. Since cell injury can cause apoptosis, invading viruses (such as the common adenovirus) prevent the cell from committing suicide (which would halt the spread of virus) by coding for antiapoptotic proteins. Accelerated apoptosis appears to be prominent in certain cell types in severe sepsis and MODS.

Every cell contains the genetic code for apoptosis, and it appears that many (if not all) cells actively maintain a network of regulatory elements which inter-

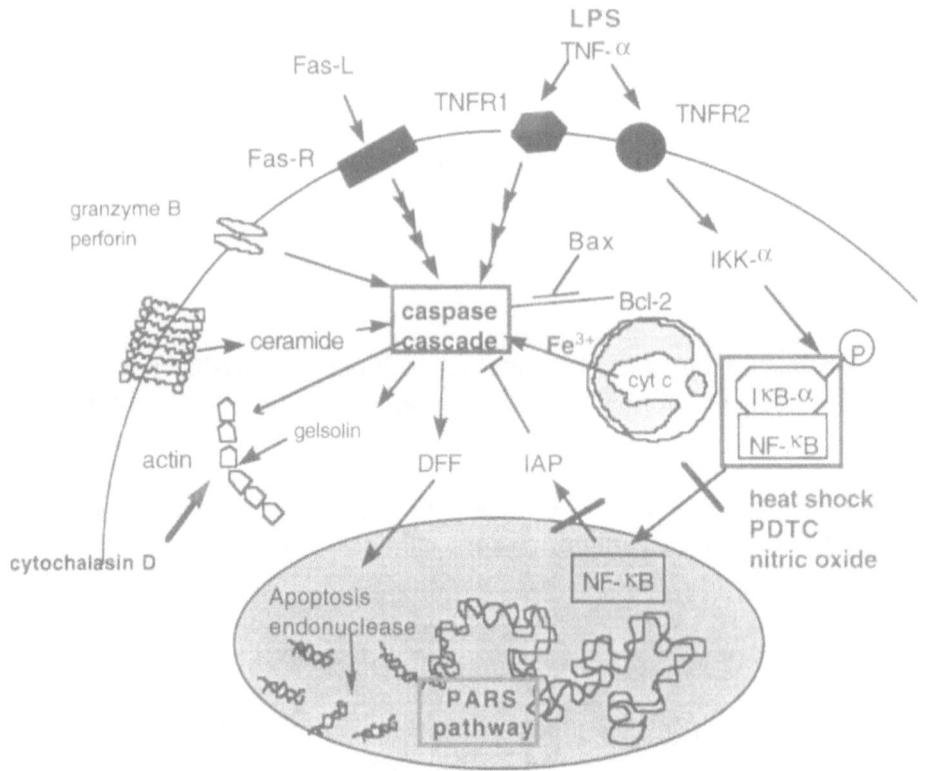

Fig. 1.

fere with execution of the code. This regulatory network has been the object of intense and fruitful study for the past decade. The field is evolving so rapidly that high resolution flow diagrams are obsolete soon after they are written. Nevertheless, the general low resolution picture of the process appears stable and sufficient for the purpose of this review. The single most important aspect of this low power view is that the regulatory network is decidedly nonlinear and thus predictions of the effect of altering the activity of any arbitrary component should be approached with skepticism until confirmatory data are provided through actual experiment.

Pertinent to this chapter are the following:

1. The redox state of the cell has been consistently recognized to play an important role in the regulation of apoptosis. In general, loss of reducing potential is permissive for apoptosis and a pulse of oxidants will trigger the process. Diverse reactive species including superoxide, hydroxyl radical, peroxides, nitric oxide and peroxynitrite have been implicated in apoptosis.

It is not clear whether specific reactive species participate exclusively in regulation of the process versus execution of the process.

2. The most important antioxidant "system" in the cell is neither a specific reducing agent (such as glutathione) nor an enzyme (such as superoxide dismutase) but rather compartmentalization of cellular processes. This "system" fails early in apoptosis as organelles become leaky during cytoplasmic condensation. Again, it is not clear whether the general failure of compartmentalization is a cause (failed regulation) or consequence of apoptosis.

3. Circumstantial evidence suggests that specific failure of compartmentalization at the level of the mitochondrion is a cause of apoptosis. In the mitochondrion, the conversion of oxygen to water can follow two pathways. The most efficient pathway, the one which initially appeared as a protective mechanism during evolution from hypoxic life, is the electron transport chain of structurally adjacent cytochromes. This has since become our primary source of energy via oxidative phosphorylation. The second pathway, often called the univalent leak pathway, is the system of superoxide dismutase, catalase and antioxidant thiols. Unlike the oxidative phosphorylation in which the destructive electron is imprisoned in the cytochrome network, the univalent leak pathway looses superoxide, hydroxyl and so on in the mitochondrial space. Substantial evolution has transpired to ensure that neither the small reactive species nor the cytochromes themselves get out of the mitochondrion. The most potent antiapoptotic protein known, *bcl-2*, localizes to the mitochondrial membrane. Besides being an antioxidant in its own right, its functions include prevention of leakage of cytochrome C from damaged mitochondria. Insertion of free cytochrome C into the cytoplasm precipitates apoptosis in test systems. Bcl-2 itself is highly regulated through dimerization with other members of its family such as *bax*, *bcl-x_L* and *bad*.

4. The caspases consist of proteases with an unusual cysteine-aspartate cleavage site. This superfamily (which includes several families with even more stringent cleavage sequence specificities) are functionally arranged in a cascade which culminates in apoptosis following diverse stresses in many cell types. Activation of this cascade has been associated with apoptosis while blockade with selective caspase inhibitors precludes apoptosis following an otherwise lethal stimulus. It therefore appears to be a common node in the regulatory web.

5. The nuclear factor NF-κB is a transcription factor activated by diverse inflammatory stimuli and by reactive oxygen species. While NF-κB activation is characteristic of the progression to apoptosis, we have shown that attempts to suppress activity following activation can paradoxically accelerate progression to apoptosis.

6. The PARS (Poly-Adp-Ribosyl Synthase) pathway, like the NF-κB pathway, can promote or prevent apoptosis depending on the immediate context of its

activation. The appearance of single-strand breaks in DNA activates PARS and the consequent poly-ADP ribosylation depletes NAD. The NAD depletion is postulated to cause mitochondrial leakage of cytochrome C and activation of the caspase cascade. However PARS also depletes the cell of ATP and thus inhibits ATP dependent reactions including apoptosis. To make the picture more complex, PARS is its own substrate.

7.   The three-way interactions among the caspases, NF-κB are confusing and complex. Caspases can cleave PARS to inactivate it. Bcl-2, which protects the NF-κB pathway and promotes NF-κB activity, also appears to protect and promote PARS activity [2]. PARS inhibition is linked to inhibition of NF-κB [3].

Pathological timing of apoptosis in MODS: animal and human studies

The mechanisms described in the preceding sections were selected for discussion because each is also thought to play a central role in sustained inflammatory states. Given the overlapping effects upon apoptosis and MODS pathophysiology, it is reasonable to ask whether physiologic apoptosis is pathologically altered in the crucible of sustained inflammation. At the lowest level of resolution, the regulatory mechanisms are ignored and we confine the inquiry to a simple ternary question: does apoptosis occur late, on time or early in sustained inflammation en route to MODS? The answer is cell, tissue and organ specific.

Delayed apoptosis

The most important example of delayed apoptosis in sustained inflammation is the polymorphonuclear leukocyte. Apoptosis is a regulatory mechanism which ordinarily acts to limit inflammation by removing surplus polymorphonuclear leukocytes from (for example) sites of resolving infection. The intense infiltrate of polymorphs observed in such diverse processes as pneumonia, hepatitis and abscess eventually have to vanish without inciting the inflammation ordinarily associated with decomposing tissue. The physiologic mechanism allowing this is the extraordinarily brief design life (less than a day) of polymorphonuclear cells following which they undergo apoptosis. The rise in WBC associated with infection and inflammation is certainly due to demargination and increased production but also may be attributed, at least in part, to a longer life span of the cells. Indeed, leukocytes harvested from patients with significant burns characteristically exhibit a delayed transition to undergo apoptosis [4, 5].

Accelerated apoptosis

Substantial experimental and clinical evidence has been obtained supporting the hypothesis that sepsis and MODS precipitates untimely apoptosis in diverse cell types.

In experimental systems which are intended to mimic human sepsis, both endotoxaemia and cecal ligation and puncture cause death in rodents and higher vertebrates. The progression of illness in these models is mirrored by progressive apoptosis in many cell types but this apoptosis is most severe in tissues of lymphocyte lineage (spleen, thymus, gut associated lymphatic tissue) and in some epithelial cells, primarily gut and (in special models) hepatic cells [6]. The severity of the apoptosis can differ somewhat from strain to strain and from species to species, but all exhibit the accelerated apoptosis versus appropriate experimental controls. The predisposition of lymphocytes to this accelerated apoptosis is not strictly due to activation of inflammatory mediators but rather appears to be (at least in part) dependent on the steroid biology of the stress response [7]. It has been proposed, but not proven, that this apoptotic pathway to lymphocyte lysis could, in part, explain the dysregulated immune responses which often accompany the descent from sepsis through MODS and death.

Systematic studies of septic humans with respect to apoptosis have not yet appeared in the biomedical literature. We recently undertook an approved protocol to perform tissue harvest in the intensive care unit immediately following death of septic patients after appropriate consent was obtained from the next of kin. These tissues were analyzed for apoptosis using several complementary methods. The data, which have been submitted for review and publication in the professional literature, suggest that lymphocytes and gut epithelial cells of patients who die of severe sepsis and MODS undergo accelerated apoptosis when compared with those cells obtained from patients dying acutely of other, nonseptic, causes such as acute myocardial infarction. The association between sepsis and apoptosis is just that, an association. Causality has not yet been determined. Again, it is tempting to speculate that the apoptotic lymphocyte depletion could account, at least in part, for the persistent immunosuppression associated with MODS. Similarly, it is conceivable that the accelerated gut epithelial apoptosis accounts in part for the appearance of toxic products in the portal circulation and stimulation of inflammatory mediators.

The apoptosis paradox

Causality issues aside, it is apparent that sepsis and descent into MODS have the potential to dysregulate progression to apoptosis in ways that are cell-type and tissue-type dependent. Given the complex interconnected web which regulates progression to MODS, it is easy to understand that subtle changes in the (external) microenvironment of the cell and in the states of the regulators inside the cell could well "tip the balance" towards delayed versus accelerated apoptosis. What is harder to understand is how cells which have identical genotypes can display such remarkably opposed responses when confronted with the same microenvironment, mediators, nutrients and so on. Preliminary work from our laboratory suggests that the immediate past history of the cell prior to exposure to significant stress may have important consequences upon the web which regulates apoptosis, and in particular the past history of activation of nuclear factor NF-κB [8].

Summary

The relationship between sepsis, MODS and apoptosis remains poorly understood. Data has accumulated which supports the hypothesis that MODS is associated with a change in the normal predisposition to apoptosis, and the alteration is cell-type and tissue-type specific. The precise relationship between MODS, which is a clinical syndrome, and apoptosis, which is a normal cellular process remains obscure. It is the opinion of the author that the relationship is reciprocal and reinforcing, meaning that therapeutics aimed at normalizing the dysregulated cellular events may favorably affect clinical outcomes.

References

1. Cobb JP, Hotchkiss RS, Karl IE, Buchman TG (1996) Mechanisms of cell injury and death. Br J Anaesth 77:3-10
2. Mandal M, Maggirwar SB, Sharma N et al (1996) Bcl-2 prevents CD95 (Fas/APO-1)-induced degradation of lamin B and poly(ADP-ribose) polymerase and restores the NF-kappaB signaling pathway. J Biol Chem 271:30354-30359
3. Le Page C, Sanceau J, Drapier JC, Wietzerbin J (1998) Inhibitors of ADP-ribosylation impair inducible nitric oxide synthase gene transcription through inhibition of NF kappa B activation. Biochem Biophys Res Commun 243:451-457
4. Chitnis D, Dickerson C, Munster AM, Winchurch RA (1996) Inhibition of apoptosis in polymorphonuclear neutrophils from burn patients. J Leukoc Biol 59:835-839
5. Biffl WL, Moore EE, Moore FA, Barnett CC Jr (1996) Interleukin-6 delays neutrophil apoptosis via a mechanism involving platelet-activating factor. J Trauma 40:575-578
6. Hotchkiss RS, Swanson PE, Cobb JP et al (1997) Apoptosis in lymphoid and parenchymal cells during sepsis: findings in normal and T- and B-cell-deficient mice. Crit Care Med 25:1298-1307
7. Ayala A, Herdon CD, Lehman DL et al (1995) The induction of accelerated thymic programmed cell death during polymicrobial sepsis: control by corticosteroids but not tumor necrosis factor. Shock 3:259-267
8. DeMeester SL, Buchman TG, Qiu Y et al (1998) Pyrrolidine dithiocarbamate activates the heat shock response and thereby induces apoptosis in primed endothelial cells. Shock 10:1-6

Multiple Therapeutic Agents - Will Individual Therapies, Each of Which Improves Patients, When Given Together, Change Mortality?

A.E. BAUE

Recent discouragement over the failure of many exciting potential therapeutic agents (magic bullets) to reduce 28-day mortality in patients has led to many diverse recommendations. One such recommendation is to use alternative or surrogate endpoints such as a reduction in severity of illness score, decreased ICU time, decreased time on a ventilator, and other evidence of clinical improvement. This is all well and good but if such an improved patient dies as frequently as do control patients, what have we accomplished? Another proposal is to use multi-agent therapy. There are many reasons why the older and more recent clinical trials have been negative. One important reason is that injury, infection and inflammation bring about complex changes and responses in the host. There are multiple pro-proinflammatory mediators with overlap, redundancy, and cross stimulation. This is followed by an anti-inflammatory response to try to control the process before it gets out of hand. The timing and variability of these processes are inconsistent. Even with similar diseases there is great variability [1]. This has led to consideration of multiple therapeutic agents for patients with diseases or injuries which stimulate an inflammatory response. I have recently reviewed the reasons why many of the clinical trials in the distant and recent past have failed [1].

Multiple therapeutic agents in other diseases

There are many human diseases in which multiple agents are required for appropriate therapy. This includes antituberculous therapy for tuberculosis, immunosuppression for transplanted organs, inotropes and diuretics for heart failure, multiple antibiotics for polymicrobial peritonitis, cancer chemotherapy and support of the gastrointestinal tract. A review of several of these disease processes will illustrate the difficulties and the evolution that occurred in therapy with the addition of multiple agents.

The development of chemotherapy for tuberculosis and its evolution over the years will serve as an example of the problems even when dealing with a specific disease process and one organism which may be typical, atypical or may develop resistance to antibiotics. In 1944 Dr. Selmon Waksman and colleagues isolated streptomycin [2]. It was found to be effective against tuberculosis in a small trial in 1945 [3] and this was followed by a large national trial in 1947 demonstrating impressive clinical results [4]. It was immediately apparent that there was a high incidence of relapse and the development of resistant organisms [5]. To counteract this effect, an agent p-aminosalicylic acid (PAS), a drug which had mild tuberculostatic activity, was used in combination with streptomycin in a trial in 1948-1949 [6]. PAS extended the time during which streptomycin could be administered without developing resistance. In 1950 a specific program by industry led to the development of an antituberculous agent which was synthesized called isonicotinic acid hydrazide (INH) or isoniazid. This was found to be very effective *in vitro* and was strikingly successful in patients in 1952 [7]. This ushered in the modern era of chemotherapy. Other drugs were then developed. The present recommended basic treatment for previously untreated patients with pulmonary tuberculosis is initial therapy with isoniazid, rifampin, and pyrazinamide given daily for two months followed by four months of isoniazid and rifampin [8]. Ethambutol can be added in the initial two months if there is any suspicion of resistance or if the patient is thought to be HIV infected. Thus, there has been a steady and continuing evolution of appropriate multiagent chemotherapy for tuberculosis. We are reminded, however, that tuberculosis is a single disease even though there are variations in the organism, typical, atypical and resistant, etc., which primarily involve the lungs initially. Much of the development of successful treatment of tuberculosis was done by *in vitro* studies of the organism in culture and then trial and error clinically [9, 10]. Also, each of the agents used in combination was effective for some time when used singly.

The development of cancer chemotherapy is another example of the complexities and difficulty in treating the manifestations and causes of human disease. Cancer chemotherapy was initially modeled after the multi-agent treatment of tuberculosis. Paul Ehrlich is said to have coined the word "chemotherapy" at the turn of the century. He used rodent models of infectious diseases to develop antibiotics. This led Clowes at Roswell Park Memorial Institute in the early 1900s to develop inbred rodent lines to carry transplanted tumors to screen for potential anticancer drugs [11].

The first modern chemotherapeutic agents were a product of a secret war gas program in both world wars. There was an explosion in Bari Harbor during Word War II. Seamen were exposed to mustard gas which caused bone marrow and lymphoid suppression [12]. This led to trials in patients with hematopoietic neoplasms such as Hodgkin's disease and lymphocytic lymphomas. This was first attempted at the Yale Cancer Center in 1943. Because of the secret nature of the wartime gas program, these results were not published until 1946 [13]. Initially, there was great excitement because of regression of these neoplasms but this was followed by discouragement because the tumors always grew back. This was followed by Farber's observation that folic acid accelerated leukemia and folic acid antagonists were developed [14]. Early therapy for childhood leukemias and Hodgkin's disease was with combination chemotherapy. There was then a long period of trial and error, observation of chemotherapy failure, and many other problems. DeVita states that, with some exceptions (choriocarcinoma and Burkitts lymphoma), single drugs and standard doses do not cure cancer [15]. In the early years of chemotherapy, drug combinations were developed based upon known biochemical actions of available anticancer drugs rather than on their clinical effectiveness. These were largely ineffective. DeVita states that the era of effective combination chemotherapy began when an array of active drugs from different classes became available for use in combination in the treatment of leukemias and lymphomas [15]. He concludes that, for multiagent cancer chemotherapy, only drugs known to be partially effective against the same tumor when used alone should be selected for use in combination. The least toxic drug should be used and given in an optimal dose and schedule. The principle of cancer chemotherapy has been clinical trials designed and dominated by the use of alternating cycles of combination chemotherapy [16]. Of course, the response to chemotherapy is affected by the biology of tumor growth. Thus, all cancers are different. They respond to very different agents. What is effective for one malignancy may do nothing for another. Malignancy is not a common denominator for therapy. Some tumors are hormone dependent, some respond to radiation therapy, some respond to chemotherapy and various combinations, some respond to both and some respond to operation with or without adjuvants. Staging and grade also have a lot to do with this. It is apparent now that permanent cure of malignancy is unusual and the malignant setting in patients is very important in terms of oncogene influence, genetic mutations and other factors.

Thus, the lessons learned from the treatment of tuberculosis and cancer indicate that specific diseases must be treated by a combination of agents, each of which has been shown to be effective individually in some way, shape or form. In addition, these processes of infection and neoplasia are chronic processes, they are not immediate, acute and life-threatening problems. Treatment can be carried out over many weeks. There are many dissimilarities between the use of multiple chemotherapy for these diseases and the possibility of using agents for the control of acute inflammation and of SIRS, MODS, and MOF.

Experimental studies of multiple agents for inflammation

Therapy for excess inflammation could require control or replenishment of a number of agents shown in Table 1. Several years ago Redl and Schlag hosted a shock conference in Vienna during which a number of speakers presented models for the use of multiple agents or multiple component therapy for the treatment of sepsis and septic shock in critically ill surgical patients (May 7-11, 1995). Aasen and colleagues from Oslo, Norway, gave a presentation based upon a study in a pig model receiving endotoxin. They used a combination of three protease inhibitors (C1 inhibitor, antithrombin III and aprotinin) together with methylprednisolone, naloxone, ketanserin, and promethazine [17]. This protected the animal against endotoxin-induced changes in the plasma enzyme cascade systems. At the same meeting Opal and colleagues from Brown University used an established infection model of *pseudomonas* sepsis and treated the animals with a combination of a J-5 antisera, an opsonophagocytic MAb, and an anti-TNF MAb [18]. They found that this provided significantly greater protection than single component therapy.

Table 1.

Therapy for excess inflammation may require control of:	
Endotoxin	Coagulation activation
Pro-inflammatory cytokines	Adhesion molecule expression
Bradykinin	Complement activation
Proteinases	Cyclo- and lipoxygenase activation
Oxygen radicals	Histamine stimulation
Therapy may also require replenishment of:	
Anti-inflammatory mediators	
Antioxidants	
Immunostimulators	

Faist presented a hypothesis for a combined therapeutic strategy which included 1) a global short-term (< 72 hours) downregulation of inflammatory monocyte activity and PMN via drugs like pentoxifylline and IL-10 or IL-13, 2) the prevention of excessive monocyte macrophage stimulation by neutralization of circulating endotoxins with high-dose polyvalent immunoglobulins, bacterial permeability increasing protein (BPIP), and soluble complement receptors, and 3) upregulation of cell-mediated specific immune performance to overcome post-traumatic immune paralysis by administration of substances like thymokinetic hormones, such as gamma interferon, and granulocyte-colony stimulating factor [19]. This is a very balanced view. At that conference Charles Fischer suggested that a combination of agents could be helpful and should be evaluated [20]. He listed BPIP for its anti-endotoxin effects, IL-1ra for its anti-cytokine effects, antithrombin III to protect against the coagulation cascade, and a complement inhibitor to decrease the complement cascade.

There have been recent studies which change some of these hypotheses and proposals. For example, Mannick et al. found that a monoclonal antibody to IL-10 restored resistance to a septic challenge in an animal model [21]. Dalton et al. found that combined administration of interleukin-1 receptor antagonist (IL-1ra) and soluble tumor necrosis factor receptor (sTNF-r) decreased mortality and organ dysfunction in animals after haemorrhagic shock [22].

Clinical studies of multiple therapeutic agents

Knox et al. used a combined chemotherapeutic regimen in burn patients in which they gave antioxidants, including Vitamins C, E, and glutamine with an endotoxin binder (parenteral polymyxin-B), a cyclo-lipoxygenase inhibitor (ibuprofen), and reconstituted human growth hormone [23]. They believe that this improved mortality based on a comparison with historical controls.

Kirton and Civetta use a three-arm strategy in trauma patients [24]. First, they block free radical production. Next, they provide scavengers. And, third, they bolster national defenses. This is done by infusing Mannitol, folate, hydrocortisone, selenium, lidocaine, polymyxin B, Vitamin C and Zantac. This is followed by a maintenance infusion of these substances and a gut formula is given enterally of glutamine, acetylcysteine and Vitamins A and E. In addition, they try to normalize gastric pH (pHi) by circulatory support. They believe that they were able to maintain the same mortality rate in spite of increased severity of injury in the trauma patients treated. They also used historical controls.

Gott et al. studied risk reduction with cardiopulmonary bypass in patients [25]. They found that pharmacologic and mechanical strategies to blunt the inflammatory response to cardiopulmonary bypass improved patient outcome significantly and were highly cost effective. They use methylprednisolone, aprotinin, leukocyte filtration, and heparin-bonded circuitry.

A review of the randomized trials of agents evaluated for sepsis or SIRS (potential magic bullets) shows that there was some benefit for patients in some of the trials even though 28-day mortality was not improved. I will review only several examples of this. There are many others.

Supplementation of antithrombin III in patients with severe sepsis did not improve overall mortality; however, treated patients required fewer days of ventilatory support, less time in the ICU, and decreased organ failure [26]. In another study, AT III resolved disseminated intravascular coagulation. Oxygenation index (PaO_2/FiO_2 ratio) improved and pulmonary hypertension decreased [27]. There was also a decreased rise in serum bilirubin and decreased need for renal support therapy. Thus, it is possible that several agents such as this could, when combined, provide overall benefits for patients. Such treatments, however, are costly. The trials are very expensive. What will be the result?

Potential hazards of combination immunotherapy were described by Opal et al. In a *Pseudomonas aeruginosa* model in neutropenic rats, they gave a combination of anticytokines, a TNF binding protein, and a recombinant human IL-1 receptor antagonist. This regimen resulted in death of all animals due to disseminated micro-abscesses [28].

There are many difficulties in evaluating a multiagent therapeutic trial. This is particularly true when we are dealing with injury, operation, sepsis and inflammation and not a specific disease process. Whether or not anyone will ever be able to demonstrate worthwhileness of a multiagent therapeutic approach remains to be determined. Certainly single agents that block various individual mediators have not been the answer.

Ideal combinations of agents

Because of the many mediators, each of which seems to have a role in the pathogenesis of excessive inflammation, it makes scientific sense to use multiple agents. If we tried to put together an ideal combination of agents for excess inflammation, what would be the components? Certainly early on in the disease process some attempts to block pro-inflammatory mediators (Table 2) should be worthwhile. Soon thereafter supplemental anti-inflammatory mediators would seem necessary.

Table 2.

Control of pro-inflammatory mediators
  Scavenging of inducers
  Endotoxin - rBPI$_{21}$
  Pro-inflammatory mediator blockade
  1L-1ra
  sTNFr
  anti-TNF Mab - to restore function
Supplementation of anti-inflammatory agents
  IL-10 - to reduce inflammation
  IL-12 - IL-13
  Anti IL-10 Mab to restore immune function
  rHDL
  Antioxidants
  Protease inhibitors
  Tissue factor pathway inhibitor
Cascade control
  Coagulation - ATIII
  Complement inhibitor
  Cyclo- and lipoxygenase inhibition - Ibuprofen
  Histamine antagonist
  Bradykinin antagonist
Control of other factors
  PAF antagonist
  Immunomodulators - Drugs, diet
  Anti-adhesion agents

Included should be control of the many enzyme cascades which are activated by shock, trauma or infection (Table 2). How many of these are necessary or important or possible to block is not known. How do we begin to formulate such an approach? What is the timing? What will be the cost? If the multiagent cocktail becomes beneficial, what ingredients are critical, some may be ineffective. What is the model on which to test such approaches? One model is the sheep model developed by Dwenger et al. with Regel [29]. These models were reviewed by Redl et al. [30] A baboon model which is in the final development stage could be helpful for multi-agent testing [30]. Would that fill the bill? Perhaps so or do we also need new "multiple models" to cope with a "two or multiple hit" theory as suggested [31]. In any case, it will be difficult to prepare a sufficient multidimensional protocol for such a study. We are told that the Food and Drug Administration in the United States would probably not approve a multiagent approach. However, all of the agents used by Demling [23], Civetta and Kirton [24] are already approved prescription drugs or are over-the-counter drugs. Will that allow them to be used in a multi-agent cocktail without informed consent? I know of no opinion about that possibility. Perhaps a trial in Europe would help. In the meanwhile, we may learn more from multiple agents in animal studies.

There are other therapeutic contributions which make good sense clinically but the evidence is divided over the worthiness of the effort (Table 3). They may help in some patients. Some of them are also controversial with some trials indicating clinical improvement and others failing to document such changes (Table 4). Some may improve a patient's condition but not decrease mortality. None of these has been accepted universally. All have active supporters and some detractors.

Table 3. Individual therapies, each of which provides some improvement in sick patients in an ICU but may not by itself change mortality

Pentoxifylline
AT III - in septic patients
Enteral immunonutrition
High DO_2 and $\dot{V}O_2$ in sick patients
Nitric oxide synthase with severe sepsis
G-CSF in septic patients
Omeprazole suspension
An in-line heat moisture exchange filter and heated wire humidifiers in patients on ventilators

For example, in a randomized trial of early enteral nutrition in patients having major operations, Hesslin et al. [32], found no benefit. However, Braga et al. in a randomized trial after abdominal surgery [33], and Bryg et al. in a meta-analysis, found that enriched enteral nutrition decreased severity of infection, length of stay, and days on a ventilator, but there was no change in mortality [34]. Immediate postoperative enteral feeding may decrease mobility and impair

Table 4. Therapy which is controversial when used in all ICU patients but may be useful in certain situations

Therapy	Indications for use
Selective gut decontamination	Acute liver failure, burns, and pancreatitis
Inhaled NO	Certain patients with ARDS
Intraoperative maintenance of tissue perfusion	Prevent ARDS in surgical patients
Protective ventilation strategy	Improved weaning
Avoiding ranitidine	Which may increase infections
Lexipafant (PAF antagonist)	Acute pancreatitis
Venovenous haemofiltration	Septic patients
Inhaled NO	Patients with ARDS after pulmonary resections
ECMO	End-stage ARDS
rHGH	Short bowel syndrome
rh G-CSF	Septic patients with neutropenia
Partial liquid ventilation	Trauma patients
N-acetylcysteine	Acute lung injury
Avoid hypothermia	To decrease mortality with trauma, and wound infections in abdominal operations
rBPI	Patients after liver resections
Enalaprilat	Improves gut perfusion in injured patients
Selenium	Improved clinical outcome and decreased acute renal failure
PGE_1	May decrease mortality in trauma patients
Plasma G1 inh (complement inhibitor)	Patients seem improved
Ventilation with a) prone position, b) kinetic therapy bed, c) rotational therapy	Improves ARDS
Lysophyline	Protects with IL-2 therapy and in bone marrow transplants
Hypertonic 7.5% saline and/or 6% dextran 70	Resuscitation particularly with head injury patients

respiratory mechanics. In general, most believe that early immune-enhanced enteral feeding is worthwhile when tolerated by the patient.

The measurement of gastric intramucosal pH has been found to be helpful in resuscitation and patient care but it is cumbersome to use and has not been adopted by all. Those who have used this monitoring technique have found it helpful in improving blood flow to the gut (perhaps microcirculatory flow) and also improving outcome. The ability to increase the pHi to normal has been associated with decreased mortality [35, 36]. Now the use of air in the balloon rather than saline has made the technique much easier.

Another example is the result of a randomized phase III trial of inhaled nitric oxide (NO) for patients with ARDS. Dellinger et al. found that NO was well tolerated with a significant improvement in oxygenation (PaO_2) (greater than 20%) in 60% of patients but there was no change in overall mortality or in the number of days alive and off mechanical ventilation [37]. This also occurred in surgical patients. One editorialist group described this as a negative study [38] whereas Zapol described the results as potentially positive [39]. He urged the use of NO in the future in patients with only ventilatory failure and no other problems. This raises the question as to whether ARDS is truly a syndrome – it is not a disease. Perhaps some diseases that produce respiratory failure may be susceptible to inhaled NO and others may not. It is worth a shot.

Mathison et al. have now reported the early use of inhaled NO in patients developing ARDS after lung resections (a more homogeneous group) [40]. Previously the mortality in their experience was 85.7%. With NO the PaO_2/FiO_2 ratio and chest X-rays improve progressively in all patients. Seven of the ten patients survived. The three that died had sepsis and none died of ARDS. Patients with ARDS who require ventilator support seem to benefit from rotational kinetic therapy and positioning from time to time in a prone position. Other ventilator strategies which seem to help include inverse ratio ventilation and permissive hypercapnia.

Patients who achieve an adequate or high oxygen transport (DO_2) and oxygen consumption ($\dot{V}O_2$) after an injury, an operation, or with an illness are said to be more likely to survive [41]. Some believe that if a treatment can drive oxygen transport and oxygen consumption to supernormal values, the chances of survival are increased. Others have found evidence to the contrary. All in all, if you are sick, it is better to have a high DO_2 and $\dot{V}O_2$ unless it is artificially increased by catecholamines [42]. It has been known for many years that patients after injury, operation, or with sepsis must be able to increase cardiac index in order to survive.

Hypertonic solutions (saline-dextran) have been found to be of great benefit in animal experiments [43]. In some clinical trials they have also been of benefit. However, the benefit has not been great enough to recommend that they be used commonly or routinely [44]. The same is true for synthetic colloids such as Pentastarch which is safe, efficient and reduces intravenous volumes required for resuscitation [45]. One place where hypertonic solutions may be of value is in patients with head injury [46]. Such solutions do not increase intracranial pressure and tend to decrease it. Whether or not the use of hypertonic solutions in resuscitating trauma patients would result in a more rapid increase in microcirculatory blood flow and improve their overall situation has not been established [47].

Thangathurai et al. maintained intraoperative tissue perfusion by nitroglycerin and fluids in high-risk patients [48]. In 155 such patients, none developed ARDS. This is a very promising and physiological approach to patient care. It requires further verification.

Pentoxifylline has a number of admirable qualities demonstrated in experimental animals such as restoring cardiac performance, tissue perfusion and decreasing susceptibility to sepsis. Thus, it should be worthwhile clinically. Two recent clinical trials suggest some hemodynamic improvement such as increased DO_2 and $\dot{V}O_2$ [49, 50]. Whether or not these changes will be enough for this agent to be used more widely remains to be determined.

Some have found selective gut decontamination to be worthwhile in general ICU patients while others have not found benefit in trauma ICU patients. Now Sun et al. in a meta-analysis, suggested that the possibility of this therapy reducing mortality is significantly better in patients with a high mortality risk at study entry [51]. Selective gut decontamination seems to be a therapy looking for the right patients. When this modality was used in patients with specific disease processes, such as acute pancreatitis, where gut bacteria may play a role, there was reduced mortality and general improvement [52].

Baxby et al. reviewed the 13-year history of selected decontamination in 46 trials. They recommended treating specific problems, patients with liver disease, burns, and medical patients after some days in the ICU on mechanical ventilation [53].

Extracorporeal membrane oxygenation (ECMO) has provided survival for some patients with severe respiratory failure who were not improved by other means. These patients would certainly have died otherwise [54].

Hirasawa et al. continue to use haemodiafiltration in ICU patients [55]. Recently they found decreased cytokine mediators and improved respiratory index and tissue oxygenation in patients with ARDS who received this treatment. Honore et al. have also found benefit from this therapy [56].

There are certainly many other experiences and therapies which could be cited and may be worthwhile. In this survey we have only given some examples and have not tried to be exhaustive in reviewing them. Are these then negative or positive studies? Some help is provided but not enough to decrease the death rate in the patient so treated. There is another interpretation which I now favor. In complex clinical situations and in very sick patients an adjunctive or supplementary therapy may help the patient but it requires more than that single intervention to improve mortality. It is also possible that such an intervention could be very helpful in a certain group of patients but not in others. If you spread a wide net for entry into a study, it may be negative because of so many different disease processes in sick patients in the study.

Conclusions and recommendations

I recommend that we study what agent or agents may help in certain clinical problems, situations or diseases such as burns, pancreatitis, multiple trauma, peritonitis, ventilator associated pneumonia. In addition, we must separate septic shock with gram negative organisms from gram positive organisms and fungus infections. We must separate ARDS patients with COPD from patients with ARDS after thoracic surgery, patients after chest trauma, and other medical patients with ARDS. Questions that will arise and must be answered are shown in Table 5.

Table 5.

Can individual agents, each of which alone reduces morbidity or improves the clinical state of the patient, reduce mortality when they are given together with other substances?

The answer!

   ☐ They don't know   ☐ No one knows

   ☐ I don't know   ☒ All of the above

   ☐ You don't know

Is it worth a shot?

   ☒ Yes   ☐ No

How do we decide on what combinations?

When?

How much?

What combinations?

   ☐ Easy

   ☐ Toss a coin

   ☐ Check your horoscope

   ☐ Have a seance

   ☒ With difficulty

Will there be?

   ☐ A consensus on the best combination of agents

   ☐ A large multi-institutional trial based on this consensus

   ☒ Multiple different combinations of agents proposed by many

   ☒ Multiple clinical trials which may lack the power for significance

   ☒ No agreement on end point

Will we focus on specific diseases and problems to determine whether such therapies may work?

   ☒ Hopefully

Will we continue to try to treat SIRS, MODS, and MOF?

   ☐ Yes

   ☐ No

   ☒ I hope not

Treating sick patients by non-specific therapy for their disease or diseases has not helped. We have learned that lesson.

References

1. Baue AE (1997) MOF, MODS, and SIRS - Why no magic bullets? Arch Surg 132:1-5
2. Schatz A, Bugie E, Waksman SA (1944) Streptomycin, a substance exhibiting antibiotic activity against gram-positive and gram-negative bacteria. Proc Soc Exp Biol Med 4:66-69
3. Hinshaw HC, Feldman WH (1945) Streptomycin in treatment of clinical tuberculosis: A preliminary report. Proc Staff Meet, Mayo Clinic, 20:313-318
4. Hinshaw HC, Plye MM, Feldman WH (1947) Streptomycin in tuberculosis. Am J Med 2: 429-435
5. McDermott W, Muschenheim C, Hadley SJ et al (1947) Streptomycin in the treatment of tuberculosis in humans. Ann Intern Med 27:769-822
6. Medical Research Council (1950) Treatment of pulmonary tuberculosis with streptomycin and para-aminosalicylic acid. Br J Med 2:1073-1085
7. Robitzek EH, Selikoff IJ (1952) Hydrazine derivative of isonicotinic acid (Rimifon, Marsalid) in the treatment of acute progressive caseous-pneumonic tuberculosis. A preliminary report. Am Rev Tuberc 65:402-428
8. Committee on Treatment, International Union Against Tuberculosis and Lung Disease (1988) Antituberculosis regimens of chemotherapy. Bull Int Union Tuberc Lung Dis 63:60-64
9. Tuberculosis Unit, Division of Communicable Diseases, World Health Organization (1991) Guidelines for tuberculosis treatment in adults and children in national tuberculosis programs. World Health Organization WHO/TB 91:161
10. MacGregor RR (1993) Treatment of mycobacterial disease of the lungs caused by mycobacterium tuberculosis. In: A Fishman (ed) Pulmonary diseases and disorders, vol. 118. McGraw Hill, New York, pp 1869-1882
11. Marchall EK Jr (1964) Historical perspectives in chemotherapy. In: Golden A, Hawking IF (eds) Advances in chemotherapy, vol 1. Academic Press, New York, p 1
12. Alexander SF (1944) Final report of Bari mustard casualties. Allied Force Headquarters, Office of the Surgeon. APO 512, June 20
13. DeVita VT (1978) The evolution of therapeutic research in cancer. N Engl J Med 298:807
14. DeVita VT Jr (1997) Principles of cancer management: Chemotherapy. In: DeVita VT Jr, Hellman S, Rosenberg SA (eds) Cancer principles & practice of oncology, 5th edn, vol 1. Lippincott-Raven, Philadelphia, pp 333-339
15. DeVita VT Jr (1978) The evolution of therapeutic research in cancer. Sounding Boards, 298 (16):907-910
16. DeVita VT Jr, Schein PS (1973) Medical progress - The use of drugs in combination for the treatment of cancer, rationale and results. N Engl J Med 288:988-1006
17. Aasen AO, Naess E, Carlse H et al (1995) Treatment of sepsis - Role of multiple component therapy. Shock 3 [Suppl]:65 (abstract)
18. Opal S, Cross AS, Sadoff JC et al (1995) Combined immunotherapy in the treatment of septic shock. Shock 3 [Suppl]:65 (abstract)
19. Faist E (1995) Immunomodulatory approaches in critically ill surgical patients. Shock 3 [Suppl]:65-66 (abstract)
20. Fischer C (1995) Unpublished discussion, Fifth Vienna Shock Forum, 7-11 May 1995
21. Mannick JA, Lyons A, Kelly J et al (1998) Major injury induces increased production of IL-10 by cells of the immune system with a negative impact on resistance to infection. Ann Surg (in press)
22. Dalton JM, Gore DC, DeMaria EJ et al (1998) Combined administration of interleukin-1 receptor antagonist (IL-1RA) and soluble tumor necrosis factor receptor (STNF-R) decreases mortality and organ dysfunction following hemorrhagic shock. J Trauma (in press)
23. Knox J, Demling R, Wilmore D et al (1995) Increased survival after major thermal injury: The effect of growth hormone therapy in adults. J Trauma 39:526-530
24. Kirton O, Windsor J, Civetta et al (1996) Persistent uncorrected intramucosal pH in the critically injured: The impact of splanchnic and antioxidant therapy. Crit Care Med 24:A82 (abstract)

25. Gott JP, Cooper FE, Schmidt et al (1998) Documentation of risk neutralization for extracorporeal circulation in four limbed, 400 patient, risk stratified, prospective, randomized trial. J Surg Res (in press)
26. Fourrier F, Chopin C, Huart JJ et al (1993) Double-blind, placebo-controlled trial of antithrombin III concentrates in septic shock with disseminated intravascular coagulation. Chest 104:882-888
27. Inthorn D, Hoffmann JN, Hartl WH et al (1997) Antithrombin III supplementation in severe sepsis: Beneficial effects on organ dysfunction. Shock 8(5):328-334
28. Opal SM, Cross A, Jhung W et al (1996) Potential hazards of combination immunotherapy in the treatment of experimental septic shock. J Infect Dis 173:1415-1421
29. Dwenger A, Remmers D, Gratz M et al (1996) Aprotinin prevents the development of the trauma-induced multiple organ failure in a chronic sheep model. Eur J Clin Chem Clin Biochem 30:204-214
30. Redl H, Schlag G, Bahrami S, Yao YM (1996) Animal models as the basis of pharmacologic intervention in trauma and sepsis patients. World J Surg 20:487-492
31. Moore E, Moore F, Franciose R et al (1994) The postischemic gut serves as a priming bed for circulating neutrophils that provoke multiple organ failure. J Trauma 37:881
32. Hesslin MJ, Latkany L, Leung D et al (1998) A prospective randomized trial of early enteral feeding after resection of upper GI malignancy. Ann Surg (in press)
33. Braga M, Gianotti L, Vignali A et al (1998) Artificial nutrition after major abdominal surgery: Impact of route of administration and composition of the diet. Crit Care Med 26(1): 24-30
34. Bryg DJ, Beale RJ (1998) Clinical effects of enteral immunonutrition on intensive care patients: a meta-analysis. Crit Care Med 26(1):A91
35. Ivatury RR, Simon RJ, Islam S et al (1996) A prospective randomized study of end points of resuscitation after major trauma. J Am Coll Surg 183:145-154
36. Ljubanovic M, Calvin J, Peruzzi W (1998) Meta-analysis of gastric pH as determinant of mortality in critically ill patients. Crit Care Med 26(1):A123
37. Dellinger RP, Zimmerman JL, Taylor RW et al (1998) Effects of inhaled nitric oxide in patients with acute respiratory distress syndrome: Results of a randomized phase II trial. Crit Care Med 26(1):15-23
38. Matthay MA, Pittet JF, Jayr C (1998) Just say NO to inhaled nitric oxide for the acute respiratory distress syndrome. Crit Care Med 26(1):1-2
39. Zapol WM (1998) Nitric oxide inhalation in acute respiratory distress syndrome: It works, but can we prove it? Crit Care Med 26(1):2-3
40. Mathison DJ, Kuo EY, Hahn C et al (1998) Inhaled nitric oxide for adult respiratory distress syndrome following pulmonary resection. Ann Thorac Surg (in press)
41. Shoemaker WC, Appel PL, Kram HB et al (1988) Prospective trial of supranormal values of survivors as therapeutic goals in high-risk surgical patients. Chest 94:1176-1188
42. Durham RM, Neunaber K, Mazuski JE et al (1996) The use of oxygen consumption and delivery as endpoints for resuscitation in critically ill patients. J Trauma 41(1):32-40
43. Moore EE (1991) Hypertonic saline dextran for post-injury resuscitation: experimental background and clinical experience. Aust N Z J Surg 61:732-736
44. Wade CE, Kramer GC, Grady JJ et al (1997) Efficacy of hypertonic 7.5% saline and 6% dextran-70 in treating trauma: a meta-analysis of controlled clinical studies. Surgery 122:609-616
45. Younes RN, Yin KC, Amino CJ et al (1998) Use of pentastarch solution in the treatment of patients with hemorrhagic hypovolemia: randomized phase II study in the emergency room. World J Surg 22:2-5
46. Shackford SR, Bourguignon PR, Wald SL et al (1998) Hypertonic saline resuscitation of patients with head injury: A prospective, randomized clinical trial. J Trauma 44:50-58
47. Vassar JJ, Perry CA, Gannaway WL et al (1991) 7.5% sodium chloride/dextran for resuscitation of trauma patients undergoing helicopter transport. Arch Surg 16:1065-1072
48. Thangathurai D, Charbonnet C, Wo CCJ et al (1996) Intraoperative maintenance of tissue perfusion prevents ARDS. New Horiz 4(4):466-474

49. Wang P, Zheng FB, Zhou M et al (1993) Pentoxifylline restores cardiac output and tissue perfusion after trauma-hemorrhage and decreases susceptibility to sepsis. Surgery 114:352-359
50. Bacher A, Mayer N, Klimscha W et al (1997) Effects of pentoxifylline on hemodynamics and oxygenation in septic and nonseptic patients. Crit Care Med 25(5):795-800
51. Sun X, Wagner DP, Knaus WA (1996) Does selective decontamination of the digestive tract reduce mortality for severely ill patients? Crit Care Med 24(5):753-755
52. Luiten EJ, Hop WCJ, Lange JF, Bruining HA (1995) Controlled clinical trial of selective decontamination for the treatment of severe acute pancreatitis. Ann Surg 222(1):57-65
53. Baxby D, van Saene HKF, Stoutenbeek CP, Zandstra DF (1996) Selective decontamination of the digestive tract: 13 years on, what it is and what it is not. Intensive Care Med 22:699-706
54. Kolla S, Awad SS, Rich PB et al (1997) Extracorporeal life support for 100 adult patients with severe respiratory failure. Ann Surg 226(4):5440566
55. Hirasawa H, Sugai T, Oda S et al (1998) Continuous hemodiafiltration (Chdf) removes cytokine and improves respiratory index (Ri) and oxygen metabolism in patients with acute respiratory distress syndrome (Ards). Crit Care Med 26(1):A120
56. Honore PM, James J, Wauthier M et al (1998) Reversal of intractable circulatory failure complicating septic shock with short time high volume haemofiltration (ST-HV-CWH) after failure of conventional therapy: a prospective evaluation. Crit Care 2:62

Endotoxaemia in Critical Illness: Rapid Detection and Clinical Relevance

J.C. Marshall, D.M. Foster, P.M. Walker, A. Romaschin

The emergence of Gram negative organisms as an important cause of infection in critically ill patients is a relatively recent phenomenon. Prior to the development of the first intensive care units, exogenous micro-organisms including *Staphylococci*, *Streptococci*, and the tubercle bacillus were the most common infecting species in hospitalised patients [1]. Gram negative infection was first recognized to be a significant clinical problem in the early 1960s [2], and by the conclusion of the decade, had become the dominant and defining cause of septic shock in the intensive care unit [3]. Investigations into the mechanisms of the profound alterations in haemodynamic homeostasis and remote organ function occurring during Gram negative infection focussed on the pathologic role of a constituent of the bacterial cell wall - lipopolysaccharide or endotoxin.

Endotoxin is a complex lipopolysaccharide, a key constituent of the microbial cell wall that makes up approximately 10% of the weight of a Gram negative bacterium. The endotoxin molecule consists of four distinct components - lipid A, an inner core, an outer core, and a carbohydrate O sidechain [4]. The latter confers species specificity to endotoxin molecules from differing microbial strains, while lipid A, and to a lesser extent, the inner core, is responsible for the biologic activity of the molecule.

Endotoxin is ubiquitous in the external environment. Moreover, large amounts, perhaps as much as 25 grams, are normally present within the gut lumen in the cell wall of organisms comprising the indigenous gastrointestinal flora. Studies performed in animals that have been raised under germfree conditions show that the presence of endotoxin is critical for normal immunologic development. The gastrointestinal tract is atrophic, with an underdeveloped mucosal immune system, and germfree animals fail to develop normal delayed type hypersensitivity, and are exquisitely sensitive to lethal infection with common Gram positive and Gram negative organisms [5]. However, endotoxin is also a potent stimulus of the non-specific immune system, resulting in neutrophil activation, macrophage synthesis and release of cytokine mediators, and activation of the coagulation cascade.

Endotoxin: a microbial trigger of systemic inflammation

Endotoxin, complexed to a carrier protein, lipopolysaccharide-binding protein (LBP), binds to the CD14 receptor of host cells, initiating an intracellular signaling cascade that results in cellular activation and the synthesis of a remarkable array of endogenous inflammatory mediator molecules [6]. These mediators, in concert, produce the clinical manifestations of systemic inflammation. Although their release can be triggered by stimuli other than LPS, including Gram positive organisms, hypoxia, or other mediators, ample evidence exists that endotoxin is a key mediator of systemic inflammation, both in experimental models and in the clinical arena.

The administration of endotoxin to rodents results in hypotension and ultimately, lethality, secondary to the release of host-derived mediators of inflammation. Antagonism of a variety of these endogenous mediators, including tumor necrosis factor [7] and interleukin 1 [8], can prevent the lethality of endotoxin challenge. In larger animals, endotoxin administration can mimic the haemodynamic profile of human sepsis [9], while low-dose endotoxin administration to human volunteers evokes a pattern of clinical and biochemical responses that are indistinguishable from those of clinical inflammatory states [10-13]. A case report of a lab worker who developed fulminant organ failure following self-administration of a large amount of endotoxin confirms the potential morbidity of endotoxaemia in humans [14].

Experimental studies showing that bolus administration of large amounts of endotoxin induce organ dysfunction and death, however, do not necessarily support the conclusion that neutralization of endotoxin will confer clinical benefit. Clinical studies of anti-endotoxin strategies have yielded variable results. Following on a clinical study showing survival benefit for patients treated with polyvalent anti-endotoxin antibody [15], a randomized controlled trial of a monoclonal directed against the LPS core polysaccharide (HA-1A) suggested that endotoxin neutralization can benefit critically ill patients with Gram negative infection [16]. Studies with a different monoclonal antibody failed to reproduce the same degree of benefit [17], while a follow-up study of HA-1A showed lack of efficacy in patients with Gram negative infections, and, more importantly, a trend towards harm for patients having Gram positive infections [18]. The lack of a rapid and readily available test to determine the presence of endotoxaemia has been a major obstacle to the determination of the clinical relevance of circulating endotoxin, and the role, if any, of endotoxin neutralization in critically ill patients.

Endotoxaemia in clinical disease states

Endotoxin is not normally detectable in healthy humans, although endotoxaemia can been detected following vigourous physical exercise [19]. Endotoxaemia is, however, relatively common in a variety of disease states.

As might be anticipated, patients with invasive Gram negative infections or bacteraemia are often, although not invariably, endotoxemic. In aggregate, 60% of patients with Gram negative bacteraemia manifest endotoxaemia [20], however there is considerable variability from one report to the next, dependent in part on the method of detection used. Van Deventer and colleagues, in a study of 473 febrile patients, found that endotoxaemia had a positive predictive value of 48% and a negative predictive value of 99% for the subsequent development of septicaemia, suggesting that the absence of endotoxin in the blood virtually excludes a diagnosis of Gram negative bacteraemia [21]. Endotoxaemia also occurs in clinical sepsis in the absence of documented Gram negative infection. Casey and colleagues found that circulating endotoxin could be detected in 89% of patients meeting clinical criteria for sepsis syndrome [22], while Danner documented endotoxaemia in 43 of 100 patients with septic shock [23]. In the latter report, organ failure was more common when endotoxaemia was present, and the combination of endotoxaemia and positive cultures presaged a high mortality.

Endotoxaemia, therefore, is common in critical illness, but its presence is only weakly correlated with Gram negative infection. In the absence of positive cultures, endotoxaemia is thought to reflect either antibiotic-induced release from killed Gram negative organisms [24] or absorption from the gastrointestinal tract [25].

A number of lines of evidence support the hypothesis that endotoxin can be absorbed from the gut when gut barrier function is impaired, or when significant changes in the composition of the endogenous flora are present. During cardiopulmonary bypass, for example, changes in gut permeability, the development of mucosal acidosis, and endotoxaemia are all evident, although increased permeability is not necessarily associated with endotoxaemia [26]. Endotoxaemia is also seen in patients with multiple trauma [27] or burn injury [28], in patients with severe acute pancreatitis [29], and in patients undergoing elective or emergent repair of an abdominal aortic aneurysm [30, 31]. Studies in children show that endotoxaemia is associated with either Gram negative infection, or the presence of a major gastrointestinal disturbance [32]. Both Gram negative bacterial overgrowth and impaired reticuloendothelial function are common in patients with endstage liver disease; endotoxaemia is well-documented in cirrhosis [33, 34], and in patients undergoing orthotopic liver transplantation [35].

The relationship of detectable endotoxaemia to clinical illness is clearly complex. Endotoxin is not invariably present during Gram negative infection; conversely, elevated levels of circulating endotoxin do not necessarily correlate with severity of illness or risk of adverse outcome. A complex biologic relationship is rendered even more difficult to evaluate as a consequence of uncertainty inherent in the detection and quantification of endotoxin in vivo.

The assay of endotoxin in blood and biologic fluids

The earliest assays for endotoxin took advantage of the observation that the administration of endotoxin to a rabbit induced an acute rise in temperature [36]. Although it was later recognized that endogenous pyrogenic activity was a result of the biologic effect of a host-derived mediator, interleukin-1, the rabbit pyrogen test was, for many years, the standard assay used to detect endotoxin contamination.

Levin introduced a more sensitive and specific assay based on the observation that endotoxin causes coagulation of a lysate derived from the circulating blood cells or amoebocytes of the horseshoe crab, *Limulus polyphemus*. Concentrations of LPS as low as 500 pg/ml were detectable with this assay, although it was noted that plasma contained a factor or factors that could inhibit the assay [37]. Sensitivity was increased to 10 pg/ml, and the assay was rendered semi-quantitative, by the development of a modification of the Limulus test that used the colorimetric detection of a chromogenic substrate to detect the coagulation reaction [38]. However, although the chromogenic Limulus assay had improved sensitivity, and became the standard assay for detecting endotoxin contamination of pharmaceuticals, its utility in biological fluids has been limited by the continuing problem of interference by endogenous inhibitors. Strategies such as heating or dilution of samples, or pretreatment with perchloric acid have partially, but not completely overcome this problem, however the inherent variability of the test, its susceptibility to contamination, and the time required to complete the test have all but precluded its use as a diagnostic test in clinical practice.

Other strategies for measuring endotoxin have been reported in recent years. Rylatt and colleagues described a whole blood agglutination assay using the anti-endotoxin agent polymyxin B, conjugated to the Fab fragment of an anti-glycophorin antibody [39]. Endotoxin or intact Gram negative bacteria induce rapid red cell agglutination that can be detected within minutes. Kollef and Eisenberg showed that endotoxaemia, detected qualitatively using a rapid qualitative assay, the SimpliRed Endotoxin Test, predicts the subsequent development of organ dysfunction [40]. Yet another approach currently under development uses the synthesis of TNF by a monocytic cell line to detect picogram concentrations of endotoxin [41]. We have recently reported the development of a rapid, point of care assay for endotoxin that uses the patient's own neutrophils to detect picogram concentrations of endotoxin in whole blood [42].

The chemiluminescent assay for endotoxin

The chemiluminescent assay is shown schematically in Fig. 1. Addition of a murine monoclonal IgM antibody to the core polysaccharide of LPS derived from the rough mutant *E. coli* J5 strain (ATCC accession number HB9081) to as

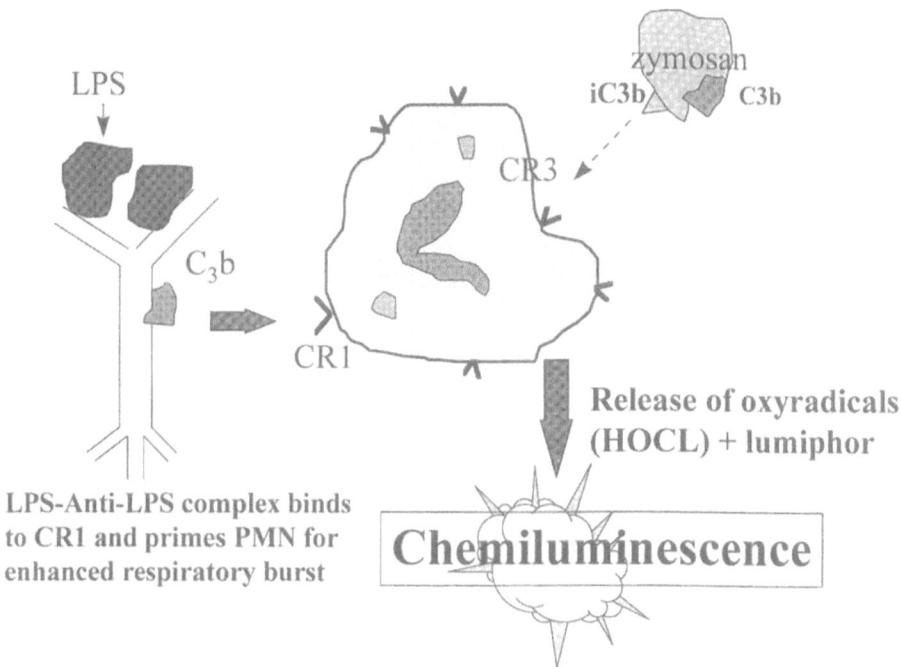

Fig. 1. The chemiluminescent assay.
Complexes of endotoxin and a specific anti-LPS antibody bind to the CR1 receptor on the neutrophil, priming it for an augmented response to subsequent stimulation by opsonized zymosan. Oxidative burst activity is detected through the reaction of a lumiphor with hypochlorous acid, and recorded continuously over a twenty minute period. Quantitation is achieved by plotting measured chemiluminescent responses against basal and maximally stimulated levels.
The assay can be performed using as little as 10 microliters of whole blood, and results are available within 30 minutes

little as 10 microliters of whole blood results in the formation of antigen-antibody complexes. These complexes, in turn, become opsonized by complement, allowing them to bind to the CR3 receptor on the patient's neutrophils, and prime the cells for an exaggerated oxidative burst in response to stimulation by opsonized zymosan. The magnitude of the priming influence is directly proportional to the concentration of antigen-antibody complex present; this concentration, in the presence of excess antibody, reflects the concentration of the antigen, in this case endotoxin, in the sample. Neutrophil oxidative burst activity in whole blood is detected as the release of light from the lumiphor, luminol, using a chemiluminometer.

Quantitation of the concentration of endotoxin in the test sample is accomplished by evaluating the response of the test sample relative to an unstimulated control and a maximally stimulated control to which 800 pg of endotoxin has been added. Specificity can be confirmed by blocking the response with polymyxin B. Since the patient serves as his or her internal control, the assay is independent of the number or activational state of the neutrophils studied. The assay takes approximately 30 minutes, can be readily performed in a rapid response lab, and requires less than 1 ml of blood to be drawn. In in vitro studies it shows broad cross-reactivity for a variety of strains of endotoxin, but does not detect Gram positive cells. In contrast the chromogenic Limulus test, it is able to detect and quantify endotoxin in spiked samples of whole blood from normal volunteers (Fig. 2). Its diagnostic utility in the clinical setting is currently under evaluation.

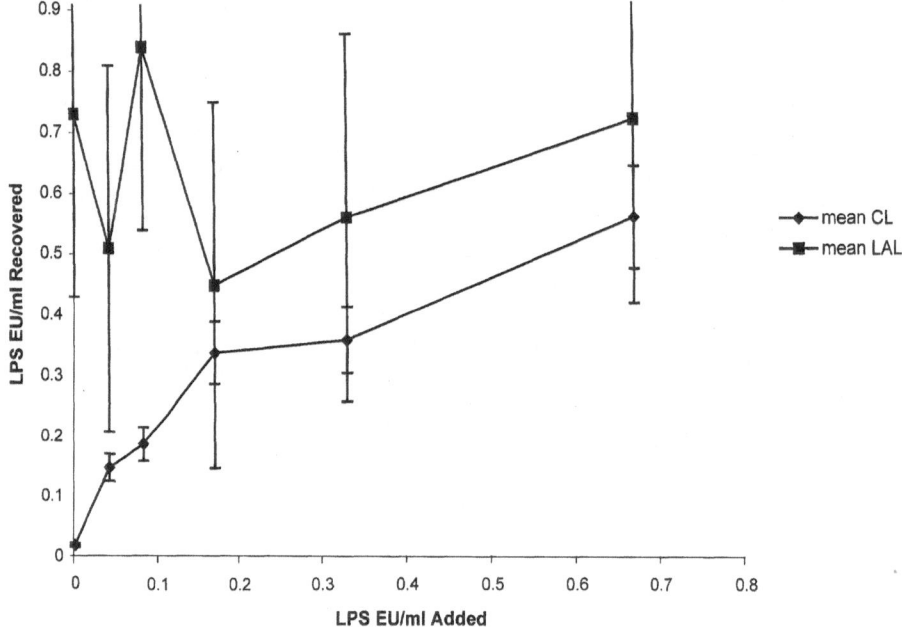

Fig. 2. Comparison of the chromogenic limulus amoebocyte lysate assay and the chemiluminescent assay.
Whole blood from healthy volunteers was spiked with known concentrations of LPS, and recovery quantified by the chromogenic modification of the Limulus test, or by the chemiluminescent assay. Inaccuracies of the former method are particularly marked at lower concentrations of endotoxin. Modified from [42].

In preliminary studies in critically ill patients, we have detected endotoxin at concentrations of greater than 50 pg/ml in 58% of a cohort of unselected patients studied within 12 hours of ICU admission. Endotoxaemia invariably accompanied invasive Gram negative infection, although it was also evident in patients in whom no infectious focus could be identified.

Conclusion

Endotoxaemia is a common concomitant of critical illness. Indeed its prevalence during physiologic stresses such as vigourous exercise suggests that the ability to absorb and to respond to endotoxin may hold some adaptive benefit for the host. On the other hand, both laboratory and clinical studies have shown that endotoxin is a potent trigger of morbidity and mortality, and therefore, an attractive target for potential therapeutic intervention. While endotoxin is of obvious importance during Gram negative infection, it is encountered in circumstances other than during such infections, and it may be an appropriate therapeutic target when endotoxaemia occurs in the absence of culture-proven infection.

The lack of a reliable rapid assay for endotoxin has been an impediment to the successful evaluation of anti-endotoxin therapies: both the selection of appropriate patients for therapy and the monitoring of therapeutic response would be facilitated by such an assay. Indeed it was estimated that the lack of a reliable endotoxin assay would have resulted in the generation of $1 billion in excess costs to the American health care system, had the anti-endotoxin antibody, HA-1A been licensed for release [43].

In more general terms, an inability to measure the complex processes involved in the expression of an acute inflammatory response has been a recurring problem for clinical trials of novel mediator-directed therapy. The chemiluminescent assay may meet this need for studies evaluating new therapies targeting bacterial endotoxin; a multicentre evaluative study is scheduled to begin in early 1999.

References

1. Rogers DE (1959) The changing pattern of life-threatening microbial disease. N Engl J Med 261:677-683
2. McCabe WR, Jackson GG (1962) Gram negative bacteremia. Etiology and ecology. Arch Intern Med 110:83-91
3. Maclean LD, Mulligan WG, Mclean APH et al (1967) Patterns of septic shock in man - a detailed study of 56 patients. Ann Surg 166:543-562
4. Sweet MJ, Hume DA (1996) Endotoxin signal transduction in macrophages. J Leuk Biol 60:8-26
5. Marshall JC (1991) The ecology and immunology of the GI tract in health and critical illness. J Hosp Infect 19:7-17
6. Ulevitch RJ, Tobias PS (1995) Receptor-dependent mechanisms of cell stimulation by bacterial endotoxin. Ann Rev Immunol 13:437-457
7. Beutler B, Milsark IW, Cerami AC (1985) Passive immunization against cachectin tumor necrosis factor protects mice from lethal effect of endotoxin. Science 229:869-871
8. Ohlsson K, Bjork P, Bergenfeldt M et al (1990) Interleukin-1 receptor antagonist reduces mortality from endotoxin shock. Nature 348:550-552
9. Demling RH, Lalonde CC, Jin LJ et al (1986) The pulmonary and systemic response to recurrent endotoxemia in the adult sheep. Surgery 100:876-883
10. Suffredini AF, Fromm RE, Parker MM et al (1989) The cardiovascular response of normal humans to the administration of endotoxin. N Engl J Med 321:280-287

11. Michie HR, Spriggs DR, Manogue KR et al (1988) Tumor necrosis factor and endotoxin induce similar metabolic responses in human beings. Surgery 104:280-286

12. Fong Y, Marano MA, Moldawer LL et al (1990) The acute splanchnic and peripheral tissue metabolic response to endotoxin in humans. J Clin Invest 85:896-1904

13. van der Poll T, de Waal Malefyt R, Coyle SM et al (1997) Antiinflammatory cytokine responses during clinical sepsis and experimental endotoxemia: sequential measurements of plasma soluble interleukin (IL)-1 receptor type II, IL-10, and IL-1. J Infect Dis 175:118-122

14. Taveira Da Silva AM, Kaulach HC, Chuidian FS et al (1993) Brief report: shock and multiple organ dysfunction after self administration of salmonella endotoxin. N Engl J Med 328: 1457-1460

15. Ziegler EJ, McCutchan JA, Fierer J et al (1982) Treatment of gram-negative bacteremia and shock with human antiserum to a mutant Escherichia coli. N Engl J Med 307:1225-1230

16. Ziegler EJ, Fisher CJ, Sprung CL et al (1991) Treatment of gram-negative bacteremia and septic shock with HA-1A human monoclonal antibody against endotoxin. N Engl J Med 324:429-436

17. Greenman RL, Schein RMH, Martin MA et al (1991) A controlled clinical trial of E5 murine monoclonal IgM antibody to endotoxin in the treatment of gram-negative sepsis. JAMA 266:1097-1102

18. McCloskey RV, Straube RC, Sanders C et al (1994) Treatment of septic shock with human monoclonal antibody HA-1A. A randomized double-blind, placebo-controlled trial. Ann Intern Med 121:1-5

19. Moore GE, Holbein ME, Knochel JP (1995) Exercise-associated collapse in cyclists is unrelated to endotoxemia. Med Sci Sports Exer 27:1238-1242

20. Hurley JC (1995) Endotoxemia: methods of detection and clinical correlates. Clin Microbiol Rev 8:268-292

21. van Deventer SJ, Buller HR, Ten Cate JW et al (1988) Endotoxemia: an early predictor of septicaemia in febrile patients. Lancet 1:605-609

22. Casey LC, Balk RA, Bone RC (1993) Plasma cytokines and endotoxin levels correlate with survival in patients with the sepsis syndrome. Ann Intern Med 119:771-778

23. Danner RL, Elin RJ, Hosseini JM et al (1991) Endotoxemia in human septic shock. Chest 99:169-175

24. Hurley JC (1992) Antibiotic-induced release of endotoxin: a reappraisal. Clin Infect Dis 15:840-854

25. Van Deventer SJH, Ten Cate JW, Tytgat GNJ (1988) Intestinal endotoxemia. Clinical significance. Gastroenterology 94:825-831

26. Riddington DW, Venkatesh B, Boivin CM et al (1996) Intestinal permeability, gastric intramucosal pH, and systemic endotoxemia in patients undergoing cardiopulmonary bypass. JAMA 275:1007-1012

27. Buttenschoen K, Berger D, Hiki N et al (1996) Plasma concentrations of endotoxin and anti-endotoxin antibodies in patients with multiple injuries: a prospective clinical study. Eur J Surg 162:853-860

28. Winchurch RA, Thupari JN, Munster AM (1987) Endotoxemia in burn patients: Levels of circulating endotoxins are related to burn size. Surgery 102:808-812

29. Kivilaakso E, Valtonen VV, Malkamaki M et al (1984) Endotoxemia and acute pancreatitis: correlation between the severity of the disease and the anti-enterobacterial common antigen antibody titre. Gut 25:1065-1070

30. Roumen RMH, Frieling JTM, van Tits HWHJ et al (1993) Endotoxemia after major vascular operations. J Vasc Surg 18:853-857

31. Soong CV, Blair PHB, Halliday ML et al (1993) Endotoxemia, the generation of cytokines, and their relationship to intramucosal acidosis of the sigmoid colon in elective abdominal aortic aneurysm repair. Eur J Vasc Surg 7:534-539

32. Cooperstock M, Riegle L (1985) Plasma Limulus gelation assay in infants and children: correlation with Gram negative bacterial infection and evidence for "intestinal endotoxemia". Prog Clin Biol Res 189:329-345

33. Le Moine O, Soupison T, Sogni P et al (1995) Plasma endotoxin and tumor necrosis factor-α in the hyperkinetic state of cirrhosis. J Hepatol 23:391-395

34. Lumsden AB, Henderson JM, Kutner MH (1988) Endotoxin levels measured by a chromogenic assay in portal, hepatic and peripheral venous blood in patients with cirrhosis. Hepatology 8:232-236

35. Bion JF, Badger I, Crosby HA et al (1994) Selective decontamination of the digestive tract reduces Gram- negative pulmonary colonization but not systemic endotoxemia in patients undergoing elective liver transplantation. Crit Care Med 22:40-49

36. Murphy PA (1967) Quantitative aspects of the release of leukocyte pyrogen from rabbit blood incubated with endotoxin. J Exp Med 126:763-781

37. Levin J, Tomasulo PA, Oser RS (1970) Detection of endotoxin in human blood and demonstration of an inhibitor. J Lab Clin Med 75:903-911

38. Tamura H, Obayashi T, Takagi K et al (1982) Perchloric acid treatment of human blood for quantitative endotoxin assay using synthetic chromogenic substrate for horseshoe crab clotting enzyme. Thromb Res 27:51-57

39. Rylatt D, Wilson K, Kemp BE et al (1995) A rapid test for endotoxin in whole blood. Prog Clin Biol Res 392:273-284

40. Kollef MH, Eisenberg PR (1997) A rapid qualitative assay to detect circulating endotoxin can predict the development of multiorgan dysfunction. Chest 112:173-180

41. Eperon S, De Groote D, Werner-Felmayer G et al (1997) Human monocytoid cell lines as indicators of endotoxin: comparison with rabbit pyrogen and limulus amoebocyte lysate assay. J Immunol Methods 207:135-145

42. Romaschin AD, Harris DM, Ribeiro MB et al (1998) A rapid assay of endotoxin in whole blood using autologous neutrophil-dependent chemiluminescence. J Immunol Methods 212: 169-185

43. Schulman KA, Glick HA, Rubin H et al (1991) Cost-effectiveness of HA-1A monoclonal antibody for Gram negative sepsis. JAMA 266:3466-3471

New and Old Markers in Sepsis

K. Reinhart, W. Karzai

Definitions and diagnostic criteria of sepsis

Sepsis is defined as a systemic response to severe infections. Sepsis is diagnosed when clinical evidence of infection is accompanied by signs of systemic inflammation. These statements have been translated to a set of clinical and laboratory criteria helpful for the diagnosis of sepsis. Ten years ago, clinical investigators started using uniform diagnostic criteria for including large numbers of patients in multicenter immunomodulatory trials of sepsis [1]. These studies provided a valuable database which helped define what sepsis means when certain diagnostic (study entry) criteria are used. Based on the characteristics of the placebo arm of one of these trials, Roger Bone published important clinical data regarding the epidemiology of sepsis (as defined by those criteria) and proposed using a set of criteria for "early detection and treatment of a group of very high-risk patients with sepsis" [2]. Since it was recognized that sepsis is a syndrome and not a disease, he coined the term "sepsis syndrome" for this group of patients.

The diagnostic criteria of the sepsis syndrome consisted of clinical evidence of infection and evidence of poor organ perfusion or of organ dysfunction. Clinical evidence of infection meant that sonographic, radiologic, and surgical evidence were sufficient in identifying a source of infection and that there was no longer a need to have bacteriological evidence such as positive blood cultures. Evidence of systemic response to infection was defined as changes in body temperature, tachycardia, and tachypnea. Evidence of organ dysfunction was described in terms of symptoms such as oliguria, altered mental status, hypoxaemia, or elevated lactate levels. Sepsis syndrome with hypotension was defined as septic shock or refractory septic shock depending on response to therapy [2, 3].

Although an important first step, these definitions were considered inadequate especially because some patients presented with "sepsis-like syndromes" without evidence of infection. To solve these and other problems, members of the American College of Chest Physicians and the American Society of Critical Care Medicine (ACCP/SCCM) sought to provide definitions for both clinical and experimental applications [4]. It was recognized that a "systemic inflammatory response syndrome" (SIRS) may be present without an infection. This syndrome was defined as the presence of two or more of the following diagnostic criteria:

changes in body temperature (fever or hypothermia), changes in white blood cell counts (leucocytosis or leucopenia or increases in immature neutrophils), tachycardia, and tachypnea. *Sepsis* was then defined as the systemic inflammatory response to an infection, *severe sepsis* as sepsis associated with organ dysfunction, hypoperfusion, or hypotension, and *septic shock* as persistence of hypoperfusion or hypotension despite fluid resuscitation.

The definitions and diagnostic criteria set up by the consensus conference however have been criticized [5]. It is felt that sepsis when identified by consensus conference diagnostic criteria would include patients suffering from common cold and community acquired pneumonia as well as patients with peritonitis or meningococcaemia. Obviously, our approach to treatment and monitoring of these patients would differ substantially. This means that the term "sepsis" as diagnosed by the ACCP/SCCM criteria does not help us direct therapy and medical attention and therefore lacks clinical usefulness. Furthermore, no immunomodulatory septic trial has used such broad definitions as inclusion criteria. Because the diagnostic criteria for sepsis lacks both clinical and experimental utility, it seems prudent to revise it.

Most European clinicians and investigators feel that the diagnostic criteria of sepsis should include signs of poor perfusion or organ dysfunction to restore clinical and experimental relevance (This would mean defining sepsis by the criteria of "severe sepsis" as defined by ACCP/SCCM). These or similar criteria were used by most if not all immunomodulatory trials of sepsis. The placebo arm of these trials have provided us with extensive information on the course of this syndrome, on the inflammatory response, on the effects of immunomodulation, in short on the morbidity and mortality of this condition [6]. Based on these clinical, experimental, and epidemiological data, it may be useful to define sepsis (at least for clinical purposes) as an inflammatory response to infection with signs of remote organ dysfunction.

Critical review of the diagnostic criteria of sepsis

Infection: Previously, bacteriological evidence of sepsis was considered important in the diagnosis of sepsis. However, this is no longer a requirement in new definitions of sepsis. The reason for this is that bacteriological evidence of infection may not develop concurrently with clinical signs of sepsis, and a negative bacteriological result does not exclude the presence of infections or of sepsis [7]. Furthermore, waiting for bacteriology may delay initiation of appropriate therapy. Because of these considerations, recent definitions require only "clinical evidence" of infection. However, clinical evidence is open both to subjective bias and pragmatic decision making.

Signs of inflammation: Common signs of inflammation are changes in body temperature, changes in leukocyte count, changes in neutrophil granulation, tachycardia, etc. Signs of remote organ failure addresses the severity of the inflammatory response. These signs should help differentiate simple inflammatory response (common cold, bronchitis, etc.) from true sepsis which warrants intensive medical attention. However, these common clinical signs of systemic inflammation are neither specific nor sensitive for sepsis. A similar systemic inflammatory response (including remote organ failure) may be caused by non-infectious insults such as pancreatitis [8], major trauma [9], and burns [10]. Therefore, these common signs do not discriminate sepsis from noninfectious inflammatory response.

Since these common clinical and laboratory parameters lack sensitivity and specificity, others may be helpful as an early marker of the infectious etiology of a generalized inflammatory response and thus allow early diagnosis and the application of more specific therapeutic interventions. Some parameters may be needed in early clinical identification of such patients, others may be important in gauging the inflammatory response and monitoring the immune status of the patient, still others may help identify subgroups of septic patients who may benefit from pro- or anti-inflammatory therapies.

Cytokines and parameters such as procalcitonin have recently drawn attention as possible markers of the systemic inflammatory response to infection.

Cytokines as markers of the septic response

Cytokines have been implicated in the pathogenesis of infectious disease. Cytokines are peptides that function as signals which regulate the amplitude and duration of the host inflammatory response [11]. Cytokines are released from various cells (monocytes, macrophages, endothelial cells, etc.) in response to various infectious stimuli and bind to specific receptors of other cells changing their behavior and defining their role in the inflammatory response. Tumor necrosis factor alpha (TNF-α), interleukin-1 (IL-1), interleukin-6 (IL-6), and interleukin-8 (IL-8) are cytokines often associated with sepsis. It is important to note that during infection and inflammation, the host not only produces cytokines with predominantly pro-inflammatory properties, it also produces counterinflammatory cytokines like interleukin-10 (IL-10) and IL-4 and soluble receptors or receptor antagonists of pro-inflammatory cytokines.

One cytokine, IL-6, has been recently used to in recruitment of patients in immunomodulating trials. In multicenter dose-ranging study, Reinhart et al. [12] used a monoclonal antibody fragment directed against TNF-α in patients with sepsis or septic shock. This trial enrolled over 120 patients but failed to show any beneficial effects of the antibody fragment on 28 day survival. A post hoc analysis of this trial suggested that patients with baseline increased IL-6 concentrations (greater than 1000 pg/ml) may have had some benefit from the drug. This hypothesis was studied in a prospective randomized study in which in addition to conventional criteria of sepsis, a IL-6 level greater than 1000 pg/ml was required for patient recruitment. However, preliminary results failed to show any beneficial effects of the TNF antibody fragment on 28 day survival. Despite this negative results, this trial is remarkable for attempting to use immunologic parameter for patient recruitment in immunomodulatory studies. Future studies may attempt to use other cytokines or groups of cytokines to identify patients for immunomodulatory therapies of sepsis.

Procalcitonin as a marker of sepsis

Procalcitonin is the propeptide of calcitonin devoid of hormonal activity. Normally, procalcitonin is produced in the C-cells of the thyroid glands. In healthy humans procalcitonin levels are undetectable (< 0.1 ng/ml). During severe generalized infections (bacterial, parasitic and fungal) with systemic manifestations, procalcitonin levels may rise to over 100 ng/ml. In contrast, severe viral infections or inflammatory reactions of non-infectious origin do not or very moderately increase procalcitonin levels [13]. The exact site of procalcitonin production during sepsis is not exactly known but even large amounts of procalcitonin released during infections do not lead to an increase in plasma calcitonin level or activity. Procalcitonin monitoring may be useful in patients likely to develop systemic inflammatory response of infectious origin. Abrupt increases in or high procalcitonin values in these patients urge to search for the source of infection: procalcitonin has been used to differentiate between infectious and non-infectious causes of severe inflammatory states. Preliminary results suggest that procalcitonin helps differentiate an infectious (cholangitis by bile duct obstruction) from a noninfectious (ethanol) etiology of pancreatitis, infectious from a non-infectious causes of the acute respiratory distress syndrome in adults (ARDS), and systemic fungal and bacterial infections from episodes of graft rejection in patients after organ transplantation. Although small patients populations and inadequate use of statistics makes it difficult to interpret the results of these studies, they do suggest that procalcitonin levels may help identify non-viral infection as a cause of the systemic inflammatory response [14].

To allow prudent use, some limitations of procalcitonin as a parameter in infectious disease have to be acknowledged. First, procalcitonin may not or only slightly increase when infections remain confined to a tissue or organ or lack in systemic manifestations. Second, although elevated procalcitonin values during severe infections may decrease to very low levels with appropriate therapy this does not always indicate complete eradication of the infection but merely that generalization of the infection or of the septic response is under control. Third, procalcitonin levels may also increase during noninfectious disease. Lastly, despite numerous observational studies, it is still not clear which cells produce procalcitonin during infectious episodes, which stimuli prompt these cells to produce procalcitonin, and what purpose do high procalcitonin levels serve during severe infections?

Conclusion

Sepsis is diagnosed when infection is accompanied by symptoms of inflammation and remote organ failure. Since symptoms of inflammation are not specific for sepsis and may be associated with non-infectious inflammatory disease, new markers are needed to allow early clinical identification and therapy of sepsis. Furthermore, new markers may help identify patients who may benefit from immunomodulatory therapies.

References

1. Bone RC, Fisher CJ, Clemmer TP et al (1987) A controlled clinical trial of high-dose methylprednisolone in the treatment of severe sepsis and septic shock. N Engl J Med 1317:653-658
2. Bone RC, Fisher CJ, Clemmer TP et al (1989) The methylprednisolone severe sepsis study group. Sepsis syndrome: A valid clinical entity. Crit Care Med 17:389-393
3. Bone RC (1991) Let's agree on terminology: Definitions of sepsis. Crit Care Med 119: 973-976
4. American College of Chest Physicians/Society of Critical Care Medicine Consensus Conference (1992) Definitions for sepsis and organ failure and guidelines for the use of innovative therapies in sepsis. Crit Care Med 20:864-874
5. Vincent JL, Bihari D (1992) Sepsis, severe sepsis, or sepsis syndrome: need for clarification. Intensive Care Med 18:255-257
6. Zeni F, Freeman BD, Natanson C (1997) Antiinflammatory therapies to treat sepsis and septic shock - A reassessment. Crit Care Med 1095-1100
7. Gramm H-J, Reinhart K, Goecke J, Bülow JV (1989) Early clinical, laboratory, and hemodynamic indicators of sepsis and septic shock. In: Reinhart K, Eyrich K (eds) Sepsis - An interdisciplinary challenge. Springer, Berlin, pp 45-57
8. Steinberg W, Tenner S (1994) Acute pancreatitis. N Engl J Med 330:1198-1205
9. Moore FA, Haenel JB, Moore EE, Whitehill TA (1992) Incommensurate oxygen consumption in response to maximal oxygen availability predicts post injury multiple organ failure. J Trauma 33:58-87
10. Saffle JR, Sullivan JJ, Tuohig GM, Larson CM (1993) Multiple organ failure in patients with thermal injury. Crit Care Med 21:1673-1683
11. Natanson C, Hoffman WD, Suffredini AF et al (1994) Selected treatment strategies for septic shock based on proposed mechanisms of pathogenesis. Ann Intern Med 120:771-783
12. Reinhart K, Wiegend-Löhnert C, Grimminger F et al, The MAK 195F Sepsis Study Group (1996) Assessment of the safety and efficacy of the monoclonal anti-tumor necrosis factor antibody-fragment, MAK 195F, in patients with sepsis and septic shock: A multicenter, randomized, placebo-controlled, dose ranging study. Crit Care Med 24:733-742
13. Assicot M, Gendrel D, Carsin H et al (1993) High serum procalcitonin concentrations in patients with sepsis and infection. Lancet 341:515-518
14. Karzai W, Oberhoffer M, Meier-Hellmann A, Reinhart K (1997) Procalcitonin - A new indicator of the systemic response to severe infections. Infection 25:329-334

From Cytokines through Immune Effector Cells to the Body

M.R. PINSKY

All forms of severe insult to the body, from trauma, burns, sepsis, and pancreatitis are associated with the activation and systemic expression of host inflammatory pathways via stimulation of the host immune effector cells to synthesize and release potent mediators of cell inflammation [1]. This generalized process is often referred to as the systemic inflammatory response syndrome (SIRS) [2] to identify the non-specific aspects of its expression. Although the initial mediators of this process are often cytokines produced specifically in response to a pro-inflammatory stimulus, subsequently a vast array of protein and lipid mediator species is expressed in a complex network that at present defies simple description [3, 4]. The initiating cytokine usually is tumor necrosis factor-α (TNF-α) which induces a generalized up-regulation of the inflammatory cascades through binding to specific cell membrane receptors on immune competent cells.

Cytokine-mediated cell signaling can alter intracellular function of the same cell that secretes it. This is referred to as an autocrine action. Similarly, cell-cell signaling can occur among adjacent cells in a paracrine fashion. Most of the known functions of cytokines are thought to be of a paracrine nature. Examples of these interactions include endothelial cell to vascular smooth muscle cell, Kupffer cell to hepatocyte, and macrophage to lymphocyte. However, if the cytokines gain access to the lymphatics or blood stream then they may act on remote cells in an endocrine nature [3]. Using this framework SIRS can be thought of as the endocrine expression of cytokine effects because it requires a systemic response from signals that normally function on an autocrine or paracrine level [5]. Some degree of systemic activation of the host's inflammatory response is probably protective in combating infection and trauma. Fever, for example, decreases bacterial growth rate, and malaise tends to inhibit additional stressful activities by the host allowing the host to conserve energy. However, if this systemic inflammatory response is sustained it can lead to remote tissue injury and death. Thus, severe sepsis may be considered as an uncontrolled form of intravascular inflammation [14]. Serum cytokine levels can change within minutes [15] and may be very different from those measured in tissues and can be different among adjacent tissue compartments [16, 17]. Furthermore, tissue cytokine levels can vary over time in the opposite direction to those in the blood. Thus, the measure of their blood levels of any cytokine or panel of cytokines may not characterize well the overall balance of the systemic inflammatory process or the direction. Furthermore, the down-regulation of monocyte activation appears to reflect autocrine and potentially paracrine functions, suggesting that the overall picture of SIRS is one of a multi-layered immunological process in which compartmentalization of the responses may be occurring between the blood stream and the tissues.

Clearly high peak serum levels of pro-inflammatory cytokines, such as TNF-α, are associated with a poorer outcome than lower levels. However, there is much overlap in peak levels among subjects with similar levels of disease severity, and levels of cytokines can vary widely over time. Importantly, peak levels of either TNF-α or other immunomodulating interleukins (IL) such as IL-1, IL-2, IL-6 and IL-8 do not predict outcome or the development of organ failure. Furthermore, there is little specificity in the cytokine response since high peak levels of TNF-α and IL-6 can be found in the blood of patients following cardiopulmonary bypass, abdominal surgery and acute myocardial infarctions. We [5] and others [6, 7] have documented that sustained elevations of two cytokines, TNF-α and IL-6 rather than their peak serum levels identify those patients who will subsequently develop multiple organ dysfunction and death. The IL-6 levels reflect better the immunological "stress" primarily because of its prolonged half life in the circulation and the fact that it has both pro- and anti-inflammatory actions.

In patients with established sepsis both pro-inflammatory cytokines, such as TNF-α, IL-1, IL-6, and IL-8, and anti-inflammatory species, such as IL-1 receptor antagonist (IL-1ra), IL-10, and the soluble TNF-α receptors I and II co-exist in the circulation and presumably within the tissues as well [8-10]. Thus, sepsis can be more accurately described as a dysregulation of the systemic inflammatory response to external stress, rather than merely the over expression of either pro- or anti-inflammatory substances. Accordingly, long ago we proposed the term *malignant intravascular inflammation* to describe this process. We still feel it describes the process better than do other more clinically related ones like SIRS and sepsis syndrome. The paradoxical expression in the blood of pro-inflammatory mediators and anti-inflammatory molecular species probably creates an internal conflict amongst the various cellular responses of injury and repair that in sustained sepsis induces impaired host adaptability. This conflict is reflected in the dysregulation of both the response of the immune effector cells to subsequent inflammatory challenges and also the resting basal inflammatory response within the tissues. This process is also known as *inflammatory-stimuli-induced-anergy* [11]. The phenomenon of inflammatory-stimuli-induced anergy describes a universal process. One common example of this process is "endotoxin tolerance" wherein prior exposure to endotoxin at a low dose markedly reduces the host sensitivity to subsequent larger doses of endotoxin. Presumably, this process is induced by anti-inflammatory cytokines, such as TGF-β, IL-10, IL-4 and somewhat by IL-1 but not by the pro-inflammatory cytokines TNF-α,

IL-6 or IL-8. Furthermore, it is associated with altered intracellular metabolism of the important pro-inflammatory regulatory protein NF-κB. NF-κB is the intracellular species that exists in the cytosol as an inactive form bound to its inhibitory subunit I-κB. Once the I-κB is cleaved the active portion migrates into the nucleus and binds to promoter sites on the genome stimulating mRNA synthesis of genes coding for pro-inflammatory cytokines, like TNF-α. During an endotoxin tolerant state, induced by prior exposure to small amounts of endotoxin, subsequent endotoxin exposure can induce the initial steps of signal transduction up to NF-κB, but NF-κB appears to be dysfunction. The active portion of NF-κB is a dimer made up of one p 50 and one p 65 monomer. If this dimer is made up of two p 50 monomers, it creates an inactive form which can still bind to the promoter site on the genome but does not allow for transcription. NF-κB dysfunction in SIRS and endotoxin tolerance reflects both an excess p 50 homodimer production, which lacks transcription activity [12], and an excess synthesis of the inhibitor of NF-κB, IκB-α [13]. The balance of NF-κB species is very sensitive to transcription rates, with ratios of NF-κB p 50-p 65 heterodimer to p 50 homodimer of 1.8 ± 0.6 conferring activation of the inflammatory pathways, while a ratio of 0.8 ± 0.1 conferring lack of stimulation in response to LPS, or "endotoxin tolerance". However, these NF-κB-related processes can only explain the down-regulation of the overall inflammatory process. They cannot explain why both pro- and anti-inflammatory activation seem to be sustained throughout the course of severe stress, such as may occur during sepsis, following trauma and burns, or pancreatitis. For a combined pro- and anti-inflammatory state to co-exist some additional processes must also be present. For example, there must be either sustained activation of both pro- and anti-inflammatory pathways or failure of programmed cell dead of immune competent cells. Programmed cell death is referred to as apoptosis. Apoptosis is inhibited by both endotoxin and pro-inflammatory cytokines. How these processes interrelate to each other and with the host has yet to be defined.

Circulating immune effector cells in sepsis

Circulating and tissue resident immune effector cells play a major role in host defense, inflammation, as well as tissue injury and repair. Clearly humoral factors play an important role in initiating and sustaining a systemic inflammatory response and in modulating the ultimate outcome from sepsis. Furthermore, local autocrine and paracrine factors alter local immune effector cell responsiveness despite common circulating levels of systemic inflammatory mediators. Still, the primary effector organ for cell injury in SIRS is the activated immunocytes, including PMNs, monocyte-macrophages, and lymphocytes. These immune effector cells are those which may induce organ system dysfunction across different vascular beds and at sites remote from the initiating stimuli. Furthermore, activation of immune effector cells occurs rapidly, within minutes, does not require new protein synthesis, and thus reflects an alternative arm of the normal activation pathways in parallel with NF-κB induced gene transcription.

Recent work suggests that cell surface receptors responsible for cell adhesion when activated can markedly modify cellular response to many if not most mediators. Thus, TNF-α may induce activation of free immune effector cells in the circulation to become rigid and stick in capillaries, but mobilize tissue resident immune-effector cells to migrate to a site of inflammation.

One method of assessing the activation state of circulating immunocytes is to measure the intensity of display on their cell surface proteins essential for effector functions. In that regard, Rosenbloom et al. demonstrated that both circulating PMNs and monocytes are activated in septic patients with liver failure [18]. This activation is characterized by loss or shedding of L-selectin, a constitutively expressed cell surface protein necessary for weak cell adhesion, and increasing display of both CD11b, a β2 integrin essential for firm cell-cell adhesion of circulating PMNs to endothelial cells, and CD35, a complement receptor. Furthermore, these changes in circulating immunocyte display correlated with both mean serum IL-6 levels and the degree of organ dysfunction but not the level of shock severity. These data suggest that clinical signs, such as shock severity and fever, are poor indicators of the internal inflammatory state. Thus recruiting patients and monitoring their response in future clinical trials of immunomodulating therapies in sepsis will require an assessment of the subject's immunological balance as well as their clinical status.

Circulating PMNs are both heroes and villains in the process of inflammation. Potentially circulating PMNs are an important contributor to both host defense against infection and the host-induced organ injury. Studies have reported divergent results on PMN activation in SIRS. Both PMN overactivity [19, 20] and dysfunction [21-24] have been described in patients with SIRS. Similarly, CD11b display on circulating PMNs has been reported to be either decreased [25, 26] or increased [27-30] in critically ill and septic patients.

Thus, Rosenbloom et al. [31] recently hypothesized that the *de novo* display of L-selectin and CD11b on circulating PMNs and their subsequent expression in response to *in vitro* stimulation to TNF-α would characterize the state of activation and responsiveness of these cells. Thus, an assay system was developed that measured both the *de novo* level of CD11b expression and the degree of up regulation of CD11b on circulating PMNs. Stimulated immune effector cells should have increased *de novo* CD11b expression while suppressed immune effector cells should have diminished expression of CD11b. On a higher level of assessment of immune competence, responsive immune effector cells should increase their expression of CD11b if stimulated exogenous TNF-α *in vitro*, whereas suppressed immune effector cells should have a blunted CD11b response to exogenous TNF-α. Accordingly, this functional assessment of circulating immune effector cells represents a method of assessing functional immune tolerance, activation or anergy. Furthermore, if therapies were to improve the normal immune balance one would expect this profile to change accordingly toward what is seen in otherwise healthy subjects or those who are appropriately coping with stress. Therapies that induced a more pro-inflammatory state may increase CD1b expression, but, based on this hypothesis, would only change functional status if they restored the *in vitro* TNF-α responsiveness as well.

To test this hypothesis, Rosenbloom et al., in a preliminary report, showed that circulating PMNs of septic humans have a constantly activated phenotype with high CD11b and low L-selectin expression [31]. Paradoxically, these circulating PMNs are impaired in their ability to up-regulate CD11b further. Interestingly, cell surface TNF-α receptor I and II density was not reduced in the cells of these septic patients. These data agree with reports of others showing that TNF-α tolerance does not reflect receptor down regulation, but rather decreased intracellular responsiveness through expression of stress proteins [32]. This hypo-responsiveness may be a consequence of multiple mechanisms. The decreased responsiveness of the CD11b adhesion mechanism may protect tissues from the influx of large numbers of activated leukocytes. On the other hand, it may significantly impair anti-microbial defenses during SIRS. Prior studies have shown that cultured monocytes from septic patients have reduced intracellular storage of IL-1b and blunted synthesis of IL-1b in response to LPS challenge [33].

Mitochondrial oxidative stress in sepsis

An obligatory initial step in the intracellular activation of the inflammatory pathway is the production of reactive oxygen species and an associated oxidative stress on the mitochondria [32]. If mitochondrial oxidation does not occur then NF-κB does not become activated. Using sensitive bioassays of "redox" state, Polla et al. [32] have shown that a specific heat shock protein (Hsp), Hsp-70 prevent this oxidative stress and blunts the inflammatory response. Numerous other studies have shown that Hsp are a basic cellular defense mechanism against numerous stresses, such as fever, trauma, and inflammation. Another group of these proteins, Hsp-23, are nuclear binding proteins capable of initiating or inhibiting mRNA synthesis. These proteins constitute a significant proportion of the intracellular protein pool, representing 2% of the resting cellular protein component and up to 20% of the stressed cellular protein component. They also minimize nitric oxide, oxygen free radical and stretozotocin cytotoxicity [35]. Hsp-70 has been shown to be an inducible protective agent in myocardium against ischemia, reperfusion injury and nitric oxide toxicity [36], but requires some initial nitric oxide synthesis for its activation. Nitric oxide-induced Hsp synthesis blunts the inflammatory response to endotoxin and TNF-α *in vitro*. These data suggest that Hsp, in general, and Hsp-70, in particular, may be important markers of anti-inflammatory modulation of the intracellular inflammatory pathways, leading to an inhibition of NK-κB activation. The interaction between the heat shock protein system and the pro-inflammatory pathway is not well described.

The initiation and inhibition of the intracellular inflammatory responses in sepsis may reflect a balance between the normal processes of NF-κB activation and Hsp synthesis. Several intracellular events must occur prior to the activation of NK-κB. Most of these events require intracellular oxidative stress as an obligatory intermediate step. It is not clear if any specific oxidative stress is capable of stimulating these responses. Several processes, such as nitric oxide synthesis and H_2O_2 can markedly stimulate NF-κB activation. These stimuli also stimulate a counter-regulatory process via stimulation of Hsp, as well as other anti-oxidants, such as Mn-superoxide dismutase. Thus, NF-κB activation may be prevented by Hsp up-regulation blunting the synthesis of TNF-α in response to a new stress [32]. Importantly, these intracellular responses need not be associated with changes in TNF-α cell receptor density or affinity which agrees with experimental observation [34]. Sustained inflammatory stimulation must deplete intracellular pools of NK-κB, as the NK-κB is released from I-κB, and then migrates into the nucleus. Thus, the subsequent intracellular inflammatory state in established sepsis will depend on new protein synthesis.

Based on these data and the associated speculations, it will be important to define better the interactions between intracellular responsiveness, cellular responsiveness and organ injury. Furthermore, identifying which patient populations benefit from augmenting or inhibiting monocyte and PMN function needs to be made prior to initiating new immunomodulating therapies with the potential to do harm. By following cellular functional markers in addition to the customary parameters during trials of these therapies we may be able to accomplish this goal. Only in such a mechanisms specific fashion can the impact of therapy on immunocyte function be discerned and related to outcome. The alternative to this approach, treatment without immune monitoring, risks exacerbating inflammatory injury or impairing host defense against infection.

References

1. Schlag G, Redl H (1996) Mediators of injury and inflammation. World J Surg 20:406-410
2. Bone RC (1996) Toward a theory regarding the pathogenesis of the systemic inflammatory response syndrome: what we do and do not know about cytokine regulation. Crit Care Med 24: 163-172
3. Marsh CB, Wewers MD (1996) The pathogenesis of sepsis. Factors that modulate the response to gram-negative bacterial infection. Clin Chest Med 17:183-197
4. Crowley SR (1996) The pathogenesis of septic shock. Heart Lung 25:124-134
5. Pinsky MR, Vincent JL, Deviere J et al (1993) Serum cytokine levels in human septic shock. Relation to multiple-system organ failure and mortality. Chest 103:565-575
6. Thijs LG, Hack CE (1995) Time course of cytokine levels in sepsis. Intensive Care Med 21 [Suppl 2]:S258-S263
7. Blackwell TS, Christman JW (1996) Sepsis and cytokines: current status. Br J Anaesth 77: 110-117

8. Goldie AS, Fearon KC, Ross JA et al (1995) Natural cytokine antagonists and endogenous anti-endotoxin core antibodies in sepsis syndrome. The Sepsis Intervention Group. JAMA 274:172-117

9. Vanderpoll T, Malefyt RD, Coyle SM, Lowry SF (1997) Anti-inflammatory cytokine responses during clinical sepsis and experimental endotoxemia. Sequential measurements of plasma soluble interleukin (IL)-1 receptor type Ii, IL-10, and IL-13. J Infect Dis 175:118-122

10. Ertel W, Scholl FA, Trentz O (1996) The role of anti-inflammatory mediators for the control of systemic inflammation following severe injury. In: Faist E, Baue AE, Schildberg FW (eds) The immune consequences of trauma, shock, and sepsis. Mechanisms and therapeutic approaches. Pabst Science Publishers, Lengerich, pp 453-470

11. Cavaillon JM (1995) The nonspecific nature of endotoxin tolerance. Trends Microbiol 3: 320-324

12. Ziegler-Heitbrock HWL, Wedel A, Schraut W et al (1994) Tolerance to lipopolysaccharide involves mobilization of nuclear factor kB with predominance of p 50 homodimers. J Biol Chem 269:17001-17004

13. Larue KEA, McCall CE (1994) A liable transcriptional repressor modulates endotoxin tolerance. J Exp Med 180:2269-2275

14. Pinsky MR (1994) Clinical studies on cytokines in sepsis: role of serum cytokines in the development of multiple-systems organ failure. Nephrol Dial Transplant 9[Suppl 4]:94-98

15. Martich GD, Boujoukos AJ, Suffredini AF (1993) Response of man to endotoxin. Immunobiology 187:403-416

16. Boutten A, Dehoux MS, Seta N et al (1996) Compartmentalized IL-8 and elastase release within the human lung in unilateral pneumonia. Am J Respir Crit Care Med 153:336-342

17. Hauser CJ (1996) Regional macrophage activation after injury and the compartmentalization of inflammation in trauma. New Horiz 4:235-251

18. Rosenbloom AJ, Pinsky MR, Bryant JL et al (1995) Leukocyte activation in the peripheral blood of patients with cirrhosis of the liver and SIRS. Correlation with serum interleukin-6 levels and organ dysfunction. JAMA 274:58-65

19. Tschaikowsky K, Sittl R, Braun GG et al (1993) Increased fMet-Leu-Phe receptor expression and altered superoxide production of neutrophil granulocytes in septic and posttraumatic patients. J Clin Invest 72:18-25

20. Trautinger F, Hammerle AF, Poschl G, Micksche M (1991) Respiratory burst capability of polymorphonuclear neutrophils and TNF-alpha serum levels in relationship to the development of septic syndrome in critically ill patients. J Leukoc Biol 49:449-454

21. Wenisch C, Parschalk P, Hasenhundl M et al (1995) Polymorphonuclear leukocyte dysregulation in patients with gram-negative septicemia assessed by flow cytometry. Eur J Clin Invest 25:418-424

22. McCall CE, Grosso-Wilmoth LM, LaRue K et al (1993) Tolerance to endotoxin-induced expression of the interleukin-1 beta gene in blood neutrophils of humans with the sepsis syndrome. J Clin Invest 91:853-861

23. Vespasiano MC, Lewandoski JR, Zimmerman JJ (1993) Longitudinal analysis of neutrophil superoxide anion generation in patients with septic shock. Crit Care Med 21:666-672

24. Sorrell TC, Sztelma K, May GL (1994) Circulating polymorphonuclear leukocytes from patients with gram-negative bacteremia are not primed for enhanced production of leukotriene B4 or 5-hydroxyeicosatetraenoic acid. J Infect Dis 169:1151-2114

25. Nakae H, Endo S, Inada K et al (1996) Changes in adhesion molecule levels in sepsis. Res Commun Mol Pathol Pharmacol 91:329-338

26. Fasano MB, Cousart S, Neal S, McCall CE (1991) Increased expression of the interleukin 1 receptor on blood neutrophils of humans with the sepsis syndrome. J Clin Invest 88: 1452-2149

27. Brom J, Koller M, Schluter B et al (1995) Expression of the adhesion molecule CD11b and polymerization of actin by polymorphonuclear granulocytes of patients endangered by sepsis. Burns 21:427-431

28. Ljunghusen O, Berg S, Hed J et al (1995) Transient endotoxemia during burn wound revision causes leukocyte beta 2 integrin up-regulation and cytokine release. Inflammation 19:457-468
29. Lin RY, Astiz ME, Saxon JC et al (1994) Relationships between plasma cytokine concentrations and leukocyte functional antigen expression in patients with sepsis. Crit Care Med 22:1595-1602
30. Lin RY, Astiz ME, Saxon JC, Rackow EC (1993) Altered leukocyte immunophenotypes in septic shock. Studies of HLA-DR, CD11b, CD14, and IL-2R expression. Chest 104:847-853
31. Rosenbloom AJ, Levann D, Ray B et al (1996) Density and avidity changes of Cd11b on circulating polymorphonuclear leukocytes (PMN) in systemic inflammatory response syndrome (SIRS). Am J Respir Crit Care Med 153(4):A123 (abstract)
32. Polla BS, Jacquier-Sarlin MR, Kantengwa S et al (1996) TNF-α alters mitochondrial membrane potential in L929 but not in TNF-α-resistance L929.12 cells: relationship with the expression of stress proteins, annexin 1 and superoxide dismutase activity. Free Radic Res 25: 125-131
33. Munoz C, Carlet J, Fitting C et al (1991) Dysregulation of vitro cytokine production by monocytes during sepsis. J Clin Invest 88:1747-1754
34. Jaaettla M, Wising D (1993) Heat shock proteins protect cells from monocyte cytotoxicity: possible mechanism of self protection. J Exp Med 177:231-236
35. Bellmann K, Wenz A, Radons J et al (1995) Heat shock induces resistance in rat pancreatic islet cells against nitric oxide, oxygen radicals and streptozototocin toxicity in vitro. J Clin Invest 95:2840-2845
36. Malyshev IY, Malugin AV, Golubeva LY et al (1996) Nitric oxide donor induces HSP70 accumulation in the heart and in cultured cells. FEBS Lett 391:21-23

Intravenous Immunoglobulins: Are They Helpful?

G. Pilz

While there is increasing knowledge on the mechanisms of biological efficacy of intravenous immunoglobulins (IVIG), their clinical effectiveness in septic patients remains a matter of controversy. At present, data suggest potential beneficial effects regarding a reduction in morbidity after IVIG prophylaxis or early treatment in selected patients. However, no large-sized controlled clinical trial has yet been able to document a significant reduction in mortality by IVIG treatment for the total population of adult septic patients.

Mechanisms of biologic efficacy

Classically, the potential effectiveness of polyvalent intravenous immunoglobulins in sepsis had been attributed to three mechanisms: First, to their content of various antibodies which can protect against bacterial endo- and exotoxins via direct antigen neutralization [1]. Second, opsonizing antibodies contained in IVIG can stimulate phagocytosis and enhance bactericidal activity of human neutrophils [2]. Third, in vivo and in vitro results have shown that IVIG can act synergistically with β-lactam antibiotics, owing to their content of anti-lactamase antibodies and their ability to sensitize Gram-negative bacteria by disorganizing their outer membranes [3].

More recently, the modulation of cytokine production of monocytes and macrophages has emerged as a further putative protective mechanism of IVIG in sepsis and systemic inflammatory response: IgG inhibits the production of the proinflammatory cytokines IL-1, IL-6 and TNF in mononuclear cells [4, 5] and also influences the release of other cytokines [6]. Besides the in vitro inhibition of LPS-induced TNF production, IgG is also capable to decrease TNF serum levels in vivo in animal models [7]. The anti-cytokine effect is mediated via the Fc-fragment of the IgG molecule [5]. IgG interferes with T-cell proliferation via regulation of the IL-2 and IL-4 production [8]. It is also capable to inhibit Gram-positive superantigen-induced IFN-gamma and TNF-β synthesis [6]. Finally, IgG contains antibodies against IL-1 [9] and increases the production of the naturally occurring IL-1-receptor antagonist IL-1ra in human mononuclear blood cells.

Clinical effectiveness: controversy and possible explanations

Despite these findings and beneficial effects of prophylactic or early therapeutic administration of polyvalent IVIGs in animal sepsis models [1-3], their effectiveness in treating septic patients remains controversial (for details, see [10]). The main reason is the lack of a documented reduction in mortality by IVIG treatment, particularly within the two largest controlled trials available [11, 12]. In fact, only one single placebo-controlled, but small-sized trial in 62 surgical patients with a sepsis score of 20 or greater was able to present solid data on a significant reduction in mortality by IVIG treatment (death rates: controls: 67%, IVIG: 38%) [13]. A second study reporting a significantly improved prognosis [14] was subject to criticism because of uniquely low mortality rates and discrepant reports on the inclusion criteria [15, 16].

The presently available information from the IVIG trials suggests at least three potential causes for the discrepancy between the promising experimental and disappointing clinical results: first, the delayed application in patients compared to the experimental setting; second, the observed inability to increase serum IgG levels in some patients; third, the use of remote and insensitive outcome measures in clinical trials, such as 28-day mortality.

Timing of IVIG therapy

With regard to the optimal timing of the onset of IVIG therapy, both experimental and clinical results favour a very early or even prophylactic administration, as it has been used in the animal models. Indirect suggestion for early IVIG administration comes from the study of Cafiero et al. [17]: in patients at risk for postoperative sepsis, already the basal serum IgG levels were found significantly lower in the patients later developing postsurgical infections compared to patients with a regular outcome. The interventional studies seem to support the prophylactic or very early IVIG administration in at-risk patient populations as opposed to IVIG use in already established sepsis. Using such a prophylactic approach, the prospective, double-blind IICSG study [11] was able to demonstrate a significant reduction in the incidence of postoperative infections in the IVIG group (36/109) compared to controls (53/112), as well as the incidence of pneumonia (15 vs. 30 cases) and the number of days spent in the ICU (2 days fewer). Similarly, early (onset: first postoperative day) IVIG administration was associated with a significant improvement in disease severity of score-identified postcardiac surgical patients at high risk for septic complications (APACHE II score of 24 or greater on the first postoperative day), compared to a historical control population of otherwise equivalent disease severity [18]. This hypothesis derived from this study is currently prospectively challenged in an ongoing multicenter placebo-controlled trial (updated score-threshold: APACHE II score of 28 or greater [19]).

Serum IgG levels

In patients with or at risk for sepsis, there seems to be an association between higher serum IgG serum levels and a lower incidence of postoperative infections [17] or even improved outcome [13]. Conversely, failure to achieve an increase in serum IgG during IVIG administration was associated with a significantly worse clinical course [17] or even survival [13]. This suggested that nonsurvivors either have a greater IgG consumption or confine IgG in the extravascular space. Whether this hypothesis – together with the putative reduced serum IgG half-live in sepsis of about 5 days [13] – should lead to serial IgG measurements and a consecutive serum level-guided dosage regimen has not been investigated so far and will have to be determined.

Study design: morbidity measures as efficacy parameters

The need for more sensitive and biologically as well as clinically meaningful outcome measures in sepsis trials is increasingly recognized [10, 20]. For IVIG, a specific marker of biologic activity seems unlikely in view of the complex mechanism of IVIG action. Rather than such a specific marker, morbidity measures such as disease severity assessment by scoring systems and their change over time could provide an information on improvement or deterioration during therapy. Conceptually, such a quantitative measure for improvement under therapy would reflect the reversal of physiologic abnormalities, which have been shown to be the most important single predictor of outcome [21]. In the case of IVIG treatment, recording changes in APACHE II scores [22] over 4 days in close time relationship to treatment consistently displayed a significant correlation with prognosis in several studies [10, 18, 23]. The use of such measures as surrogate study endpoints in controlled treatment trials in sepsis as an indicator of therapeutic efficacy seems reasonable and has already been accomplished in the recent multicenter, randomized, prospective, placebo-controlled, double-blind SBITS trial (Score-Based Immunoglobulin Therapy of Sepsis), which has included 653 patients [12]. The prepublished concept of this study [10] included a priori the use of score-quantified changes in disease severity as prospectively defined secondary study endpoints. Another recently published finding, that early IVIG application mitigates the severity of critical illness polyneuropathy following sepsis [24] might provide a further morbidity marker for future trials. Similarly important, it emphasises the need to continue the efforts for a better pathophysiologic understanding of the target organ systems involved and mechanisms of biologic efficacy in potentially beneficial effects of IVIG in sepsis.

References

1. Pollack M (1983) Antibody activity against Pseudomonas aeruginosa in immune globulins prepared for intravenous use in humans. J Infect Dis 147:1090-1098
2. Fischer GW, Hunter KW, Hemming VG et al (1983) Functional antibacterial activity of a human intravenous immunoglobulin preparation: In vitro and in vivo studies. Vox Sang 44: 296-299
3. Dalhoff A (1985) In vitro and in vivo effect of immunoglobulin G on the integrity of bacterial membranes. Infection 13[Suppl 2]:S185-S191
4. Andersson JP, Andersson UG (1990) Human intravenous immunoglobulin modulates monokine production in vitro. Immunology 71:372-376
5. Horiuchi A, Abe Y, Miyake M et al (1993) Natural human IgG inhibits the production of tumor necrosis factor and interleukin-1 alpha through the Fc portion. Surgery Today 23: 241-245
6. Skansen-Saphir U, Andersson J, Bjork L et al (1994) Lymphokine production induced by streptococcal pyrogenic exotoxin-A is selectively down-regulated by pooled human IgG. Eur J Immunol 24:916-922
7. Shimozato T, Iwata M, Tamura N (1990) Suppression of tumor necrosis factor alpha production by a human immunoglobulin preparation for intravenous use. Infect Immun 58: 1384-1390
8. Amran D, Renz H, Lack G et al (1994) Suppression of cytokine-dependent human T-cell proliferation by intravenous immunoglobulin. Clin Immunol Immunpathol 73:180-186
9. Svenson M, Hansen MB, Bendtzen K (1993) Binding of cytokines to pharmaceutically prepared human immunoglobulin. J Clin Invest 92:2533-2539
10. Pilz G, Fateh-Moghadam S, Viell B et al (1993) Supplemental immunoglobulin therapy in sepsis and septic shock - comparison of mortality under treatment with polyvalent i.v. immunoglobulin versus placebo. Protocol of a multicenter, randomized, prospective, double-blind trial. Theor Surg 8:61-83
11. The Intravenous Immunoglobulin Collaborative Study Group (1992) Prophylactic intravenous administration of standard immune globulin as compared with core-lipopolysaccharide immune globulin in patients at high risk of postsurgical infection. N Engl J Med 327:234-240
12. Werdan K, Pilz G, and the SBITS Study Group (1997) Polyvalent immune globulins. Shock 7 [Suppl 1]:5
13. Dominioni L, Dionigi R, Zanello M et al (1991) Effects of high-dose IgG on survival of surgical patients with sepsis scores of 20 or greater. Arch Surg 126:236-240
14. Schedel I, Dreikhausen U, Nentwig B et al (1991) Treatment of Gram-negative septic shock with an immunoglobulin preparation: a prospective, randomized clinical trial. Crit Care Med 19:1104-1113
15. Werdan K, Pilz G (1992) Treatment of Gram-negative septic shock with an immunoglobulin. Letter to the Editor. Crit Care Med 20:1364-1365
16. Wortel CH, Dellinger P (1993) Treatment of Gram-negative septic shock with an immunoglobulin preparation: a prospective, randomized clinical trial. Letter to the Editor. Crit Care Med 21:163-165
17. Cafiero F, Gipponi M, Bonalumi U et al (1992) Prophylaxis of infection with intravenous immunoglobulins plus antibiotic for patients at risk for sepsis undergoing surgery for colorectal cancer: Results of a randomized, multicenter clinical trial. Surgery 112:24-31
18. Pilz G, Kreuzer E, Kaab S et al (1994) Early sepsis treatment with immunoglobulins after cardiac surgery in score-identified high-risk patients. Chest 105:76-82 (Errata in 105:1924)
19. Kuhn C, Muller-Werdan U, Pilz G et al (1997) Early risk stratification of patients after cardiac surgery using extracorporeal circulation - identification of an escalating systemic inflammatory response syndrome. Eur Heart J 18[Suppl]:585
20. Petros AJ, Marshall JC, van Saene HKF (1995) Should morbidity replace mortality as an endpoint for clinical trials in intensive care? Lancet 345:369-371

21. Knaus WA, Wagner DP, Zimmerman JE et al (1993) Variations in mortality and length of stay in intensive care units. Ann Intern Med 118:753-761
22. Knaus WA, Draper EA, Wagner DP et al (1985) APACHE II: A severity of disease classification system. Crit Care Med 13:818-829
23. Pilz G, Appel R, Kreuzer E et al (1997) Comparison of early IgM-enriched immunoglobulin vs polyvalent IgG administration in score-identified postcardiac surgical patients at high risk for sepsis. Chest 111:419-426
24. Mohr M, Englisch L, Roth A et al (1997) Effects of early treatment with immunoglobulin on critical illness polyneuropathy following multiple organ failure and gram-negative sepsis. Intensive Care Med 23:1144-1149

CLINICAL ASPECTS OF SPLANCHNIC ISCHAEMIA AND OXYGEN METABOLISM

Is Splanchnic Perfusion a Critical Problem in Sepsis?

M. Poeze, J.W.M. Greve, G. Ramsay

For years variations in splanchnic perfusion have been known to occur in critically ill patients, since they have an important role in the control of systemic blood pressure and volume. In patients with an acute hypovolaemia, due to haemorrhage, maintaining an adequate perfusion through the splanchnic system is considered secondary to maintaining perfusion through vital organs [1]. In previous decades little attention, therefore, was paid to maintaining an adequate splanchnic perfusion in these patients.

Recently however, attention focused on the influences of regional hypoperfusion, since numerous studies indicated that the splanchnic region contributed to the development of multiple organ failure (MOF) on the intensive care [2-4]. Moreover, the splanchnic region is the largest lymphoid organ in the body and is considered to have an important role in the immune response of a patient with sepsis and multiple organ failure [5, 6]. The gut provides a large absorptive area for absorption of nutritients [7]. However, it also functions as an important barrier against bacteria and bacterial products [8].

Although an inadequate perfusion in the splanchnic area seems to be associated with a deterioration in these functions, the exact mechanism behind the association between MOF and the regional perfusion disturbances is poorly understood [9]. Several mechanisms have been proposed as an explanation for this association. The presence of tissue hypoxia [10], bacterial translocation [11] and increased intestinal permeability [12] have all been associated with the development of MOF, although a debate is still going on whether these mechanisms are the cause or just an epiphenomenon of the underlying condition [13]. The occurrence of ischaemia/reperfusion of the gut may contribute, but these assumptions were mainly drawn from experimental studies. Moreover, evidence from clinical studies have been limited by the comparing of data obtained in patients with a variety of conditions.

This chapter will provide a review of the physiological basis of splanchnic perfusion, and evidence from experimental and clinical studies concerning perfusion disturbances in septic and pre-septic conditions.

Physiology of splanchnic perfusion and oxygenation

The splanchnic organs include the liver, stomach, spleen, pancreas, and small and large intestines. The upper gastro-intestinal tract is supplied through the celiac trunk. The main branches from the celiac trunk supply the liver (common hepatic artery), stomach (common hepatic, splenic, and left gastric artery), duodenum (common hepatic artery), spleen (splenic artery), and pancreas (common hepatic and splenic artery). In general, the lower intestinal tract draws its blood supply from two main arteries: the superior and inferior mesenteric arteries. Anatomical variations in this scheme are common, such that the duodenum and pancreas are usually also supplied by the superior mesenteric artery.

The venous efflux from the gastro-intestinal tract runs through the hepatic veins. The liver receives blood both from the hepatic artery, and the portal vein (±70%), which drains blood from all the other splanchnic organs.

Recent studies on splanchnic flow have focussed, not on the macrocirculation, but on intestinal villus perfusion. The villi and intestinal mucosa are supplied by a complex network of vessels. Blood is supplied normally by a central arteriole and is drained by venules surrounding the central arteriole. Using a counter flow mechanism the exchange of oxygen from the artery to the vein is facilitated. However, this countercurrent exchange of oxygen makes the tip of the villus more susceptible to hypoxic or hypoperfusional events. Moreover, the arterioles that supply the villus branch off at right angles and the presence of pre-capillary sphincters renders the mucosal layer susceptible to an absolute or relative oxygen lack during low-flow conditions and septic shock.

The splanchnic blood supply is influenced by various factors, such as variations in splanchnic metabolism, feeding and systemic perfusion [9].The sympathetic nervous control is also an important factor of variations in gut blood flow, through modulation of the degree of vasoconstriction of the arterioles that supply the villus. This sympathetic nervous control can be influenced not only by central nervous stimulation, but also by endogenous circulating catecholamines. In this chapter the influences of the latter will be discussed. The vessels supplying the splanchnic region respond to α-adrenergic stimulation with vasodilatation and to β-adrenergic stimulation with vasoconstriction [9].

The exogenous cathecholamines administered on the ICU to critically ill patients all have different effects on the splanchnic perfusion, depending on the receptor profile of the agent.

Methods for assessing splanchnic perfusion

In the past decades several techniques have been developed clinically in order to give an estimate of the hepatosplanchnic perfusion. Some of these techniques give an estimate of the perfusion of all hepatosplanchnic organs, while others measure perfusion more locally. The techniques available are ICG-flow measurement, aminopyrine clearance, Laser Doppler velocimetry, and gastric intra-mucosal pH measurement.

Most clinical experience has been obtained using ICG-dilution and gastric tonometry. The Fick principle is used for measuring total hepatosplanchnic blood flow, using the rapid uptake of ICG by the liver [14]. Previously, hepatic catheterization was necessary for the measurement, but more recently catheteri-zation of the femoral artery was shown to be sufficient for measuring hepatos-planchnic perfusion using the ICG dilution-COLD system [15]. Although gas-tric tonometry does not always correlate with measurements of ICG-flow [16], both parameters are able to identify the patients at risk of multiple organ failure. The presence of gastric intramucosal acidosis as judged by tonometry probably indicates locally disturbed perfusion [17]. However, through shunting of blood, the total hepatosplanchnic flow as measured by ICG-dilution may be preserved or even increased [16]. In a study by Maynard et al. gastric pHi and ICG-meas-ured total hepatosplanchnic flow were compared as predictor of mortality. Gas-tric pH assessment could better predict the occurrence of death than ICG-dilu-tion [18].

The method of measuring splanchnic perfusion by aminopyrine clearance is based on the permeability of the gastric mucosa to aminopyrine [19]. In an un-ionized phase aminopyrine can freely diffuse through the mucosa. In contrast to the hydrogen-ions of plasma, the hydrogen-ions of gastric juice causes an ion-ization of the aminopyrine, which results in a trapping of the aminopyrine in the gastric lumen. However, the experience with this technique in septic patients has been limited.

Transoesophageal duplex Doppler velocimetry can be used to measure flow in separate vessels sequentially, such as the celiac artery and the superior mesenteric artery [20]. In a study by Dalton et al. duplex ultrasound in humans was able to closely monitor decreasing splanchnic perfusion during small vol-ume haemorrhage [20]. However, experience is still limited with this technique and it requires expertise.

Splanchnic perfusion in experimental sepsis

In experimental studies an increase in total hepatosplanchnic blood flow is ob-served during sepsis. However, the metabolic demand increases even more than the increase in flow, resulting in an inadequate tissue oxygenation. This inade-quate tissue perfusion is complicated by an impaired microvascular function in sepsis and thereby impaired flow regulation in the gut [9], causing inhomoge-nous flow distribution of the microcirculation [21].

The findings concerning the splanchnic perfusion, however, are highly species-dependent. In a hyperdynamic normotensive model in the pig a decrease in mesenteric blood flow is seen [22]. In rats and rabbits hepatosplanchnic blood flow increases in response to the endotoxic challenge [22]. However, when the challenge is massive and acute, mesenteric blood flow can also decrease in these models. Turnbull showed that endotoxic challenge decreased superior mesenteric artery blood flow temporarely, but that this decrease was sustained when the endotoxic shock was preceded by haemorrhagic shock [23]. The adequacy of resuscitation and the magnitude of the challenge seem to determine the mesenteric blood flow in animal sepsis.

Fink et al. showed that in a porcine model of endotoxaemia the decreased mesenteric blood flow was accompanied by intestinal mucosal acidosis [24]. Restoration of the mesenteric perfusion could be achieved by treating the animals with fluids and dobutamine, but complete recovery of mucosal acidosis did not occur. They concluded that this must be due to the disturbed local microvascular flow regulation induced by endotoxin. In other studies the use of dopexamine and dopamine could also reverse the mesenteric blood flow and dopexamine could restore gastric mucosal acidosis [9, 25].

Endothelial dysfunction during sepsis

The pathophysiology behind this dysregulation of microvascular control is not completely understood. During sepsis in animals both functional and anatomical microcirculatory abnormalities, with decreased capillary density [26] and increased flow heterogeneity [27] are present in the splanchnic endothelium [28, 29]. These changes are probably related to defects in the endothelium. Until recently, the endothelium was thought to be passive and metabolically unimportant during sepsis. Now it is known that the endothelium plays an integral part in the acute inflammatory response (Fig. 1). Among many other inflammatory mediators, it releases nitric oxide, previously known as endothelium-derived relaxing factor [30]. This induces a vascular relaxation by activating soluble guanylate cyclase, which in turn causes an increase in intracellular cyclic GMP causing vascular smooth muscle to relax [31]. In patients with sepsis the level of nitric oxide in plasma is significantly increased, which causes a loss in peripheral vascular tone [32]. Other data suggest that other factors, besides nitric oxide, must play a role in the vascular responsiveness in the early phases after an endotoxic insult [31].

During sepsis the splanchnic endothelium is not only activated to release inflammatory mediators, but is also damaged by endotoxin. Endotoxins, and endotoxin-induced cytokines can alter the glucose metabolism and pyruvate dehydrogenase (PDH) activation [33]. During upregulation of the glucose transport into the cells and inhibition of PDH activity due to endotoxin, the lactate production is increased with a net release of protons. Electrons derived from oxidation occurring within the citric acid cycle are passed down the respiratory chain involving several enzymatic electron acceptors, including cytochrome aa_3. Under normal conditions the protons can be pumped through the inner membrane of the mitochondrium against their concentration gradient enabled by the reactions in the respiratory chain. However, during sepsis cytochrome aa_3 was

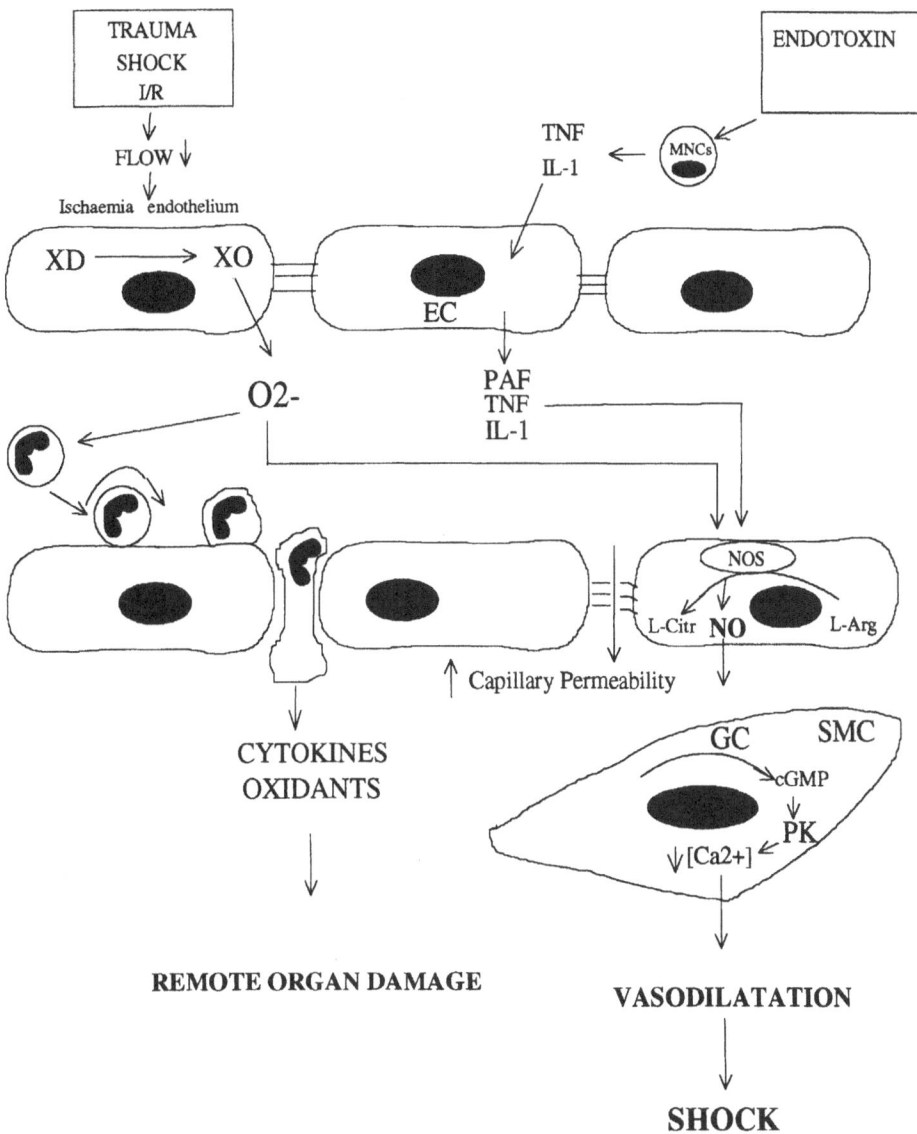

Fig. 1. Pathophysiology of vasoplegia in sepsis

shown to be severely dysfunctional, causing a loss of respiratory control (uncoupling of electron transfer and ATP formation) [34]. This will inhibit the synthesis of ATP, thereby reducing cell viability. The extent of these changes depend on the tissue examined. Schaefer et al. showed that the fall in cytochrome aa_3 activity caused by endotoxin was apparent in the gut, but did not occur in the brain [35]. Interestingly, despite the fact that the reduction in gut cytochrome aa_3 function only occurred in the presence of endotoxin-induced reduction of splanchnic perfusion, this reduction of cytochrome aa_3 was not prevented when the fall in superior mesenteric blood flow was prevented [35].

These data indicate that in animal studies endotoxin induces perfusion abnormalities in the gut. Endotoxin induces damage to the splanchnic endothelium, due to disturbed metabolic functioning of the endothelial cells.

Splanchnic perfusion in clinical sepsis

In contrast to the studies by Fink et al., in patients with sepsis splanchnic blood flow is higher than normal [36]. However, in these studies an increase in oxygen consumption was found not matched by the increase in flow. This causes a mismatching of oxygen delivery and oxygen consumption in the hepatosplanchnic area, despite increased oxygen extraction [36, 37]. Especially the increased demand in patients with sepsis, with increased lactate and amino acid uptake, seems to be a hallmark of the changes in perfusion. Correction of hypotension or hypovolaemia in these patients can increase the splanchnic blood flow to a higher level, indicating that fluid therapy in patients with sepsis can increase perfusion to a level more equal to the oxygen consumption requirements [38]. However, the mismatch between oxygen delivery and consumption appears to be sustained despite increased fluid or vasopressor therapy.

In patients with sepsis pHi is significantly decreased compared to critically ill patients without sepsis [22]. The presence of a lowered pHi in patients with sepsis predicts poor outcome [39].

The relation between total splanchnic blood flow and gastric intramucosal hypoperfusion is not clear yet. Dopamine could increase total splanchnic blood flow in septic patients, but decreased pHi [9] (Table 1). Olson et al. also reported that dopamine could not increase pHi [40]. Norepinephrine had variable effects on total hepatosplanchnic blood flow, but could increase pHi [41]. However, Ruokonen could not find an increased splanchnic flow in patients with sepsis

Table 1. Effects of vasopressors on measurements of splanchnic perfusion in clinical sepsis and pre-septic conditions

Vasopressor	Sepsis	Non-sepsis
Dopamine	↑ TSF =↓ pHi	↑ TSF
Dobutamine	↑ pHi	↑ TSF
Dopexamine	?	↑ TSF ↑ pHi
Norepinephrine	↑↓ TSF	?
Epinephrine	↓ pHi	?

TSF, total splanchnic blood flow; pHi, gastric intramucosal pH treated with norepinephrine, as measured by ICG dilution [42]. In a nice study by Levy et al. pHi could be restored by using norepinephrine-dobutamine combination, whereas epinephrine decreased pHi, despite similar effects on global haemodynamics in both treatment regimes [43]. In a study by Gutierrez et al. dobutamine could reverse intramucosal acidosis in septic patients [44]. From these studies it can be concluded that the various vasoactive agents have different effects on splanchnic perfusion in septic patients. The effects on mucosal blood flow are difficult to predict in individual patients and can be different from the effects on total hepatosplanchnic blood flow [45].

Splanchnic perfusion in experimental non-endotoxaemic conditions

Splanchnic perfusion during shock or hypovolaemia induces a decrease in splanchnic blood flow and intramucosal acidosis [46]. The vasoregulatory control of splanchnic perfusion is preserved during a long period in these conditions. Thus, this decreased flow and the occurrence of acidosis is due to splanchnic vasoconstriction. Bitterman et al. showed that superior mesenteric blood flow could be increased with hypertonic saline after haemorrhagic shock [47]. However, Oud et al. showed that prompt and adequate restoration of the systemic blood pressure after resuscitation failed to restore gastric intramucosal pHi [48]. This prolonged intramucosal acidosis and mucosal hypoperfusion [17] increases the risk of splanchnic hypoxia, with an increased risk on the development of an ongoing inflammatory response with neutrophil activation [49] and xanthine oxidase release and subsequent organ damage.

In contrast to experimental sepsis models, the number of studies using modulation of splanchnic perfusion with vasoactive agents are scarce in these pre-septic conditions. Johnson et al. showed that portal flow is restored by dopamine after a significant reduction in flow by non-bacterial acute lung injury and the use of PEEP [50]. In dogs the use of dopamine after cardiopulmonary bypass could only increase gastric blood flow, but not the intestinal blood flow [51]. In contrast, dobutamine could elevate blood flow of most visceral organs in this study. In a study by Chintala et al. dopexamine restored splanchnic perfusion after haemorrhage to 80-100% of baseline level [52]. Unfortunately, in this study intramucosal pHi was not measured, so no data were available about the effects of dopexamine in experimental non-endotoxaemic models on mucosal blood flow.

Splanchnic perfusion in clinical pre-septic studies

In contrast to the experimental studies, numerous clinical studies have been performed in modulating splanchnic perfusion with vasoactive substances during pre-septic (low-flow) conditions. Gastric intramucosal pH decreased significant-ly in response to major abdominal surgery in the patients who developed com-plications [53] and this correlated well with systemic levels of inflammatory mediators in the blood. This decreased pHi is also seen in patients undergoing orthotopic liver transplantation, cardiopulmonary bypass, and in patients with acute circulatory failure and small volume haemorrhage [20, 54-57].

As in experimental models reversal of systemic perfusion abnormalities after transient hypovolaemia showes a protracted reversal of pHi [58]. Since vasoreg-ulation remains functional in hypovolaemia (without the influences of endotox-aemia), occult systemic hypovolaemia after resuscitation are compensated for a prolonged period by increased splanchnic vasoconstriction and reduced splanch-nic blood flow. Restoring this occult hypovolaemia by administering fluids has been shown to improve splanchnic perfusion and outcome [59]. However, pro-longed periods of splanchnic hypoperfusion will eventually lead to tissue dam-age and organ failure, as will severe hypoperfusion combined with severe acute hypovolaemia, especially when combined with tissue injury, such as in trauma patients. The use of vasopressors may be useful in these patients, with adequate monitoring.

In a study by Ruokonen dobutamine could restore splanchnic oxygenation in parallel with improvement in global oxygenation in patients with low cardiac output syndrome after cardiac surgery [60] (Table 1). This effect of dobutamine could be confirmed in patients undergoing liver resection [61]. In a study in liv-er transplant patients dopamine, dobutamine, and dopexamine could all increase total hepatosplanchnic flow and oxygen supply [62]. In a recent study, dopex-amine seemed to be able to increase gastric intramucosal pH in high-risk surgi-cal patients with a low pre-operative pHi, independently from global oxygen de-livery [unpublished data].

The effects of norepinephrine and epinephrine on splanchnic perfusion have not been studied at present in patients with non-septic conditions.

Summary

From this review it seems that splanchnic perfusion plays an important role in the pathophysiology of sepsis and organ failure. Although the exact mechanism is not clear at present, studies have indicated that the splanchnic region is espe-cially vulnerable to the perfusion abnormalities seen in complications in surgi-cal and critically ill patients. Monitoring perfusion in this area may therefore be a good marker for occult hypovolaemia and hypoperfusion. There are indeed in-dications that monitoring regional perfusion is more precise in predicting ad-verse outcome than monitoring global perfusion. Aiming at improving regional perfusion disturbance seems, at present, to be a good approach at preventing multiple organ failure. The use of vasopressor therapy has been investigated most extensively in these conditions. From the studies published so far, vasopressor therapy in septic patients seems to be ineffective in modulating outcome, probably because they do not treat the vasoplegia accompanying sepsis. These changes in vasoreactivity have not yet occurred or only to a limited extent in pre-septic conditions, when the disturbance of splanchnic perfusion has not been present for a prolonged period or was not accompanied with extensive tissue injury. Increasing splanchnic perfusion with fluids and vasopressors may therefore reduce the complications related to impaired splanchnic perfusion. Dopexamine seems to have this effect independently from effects on global oxygenation. More studies are needed to investigate in detail the effects of vasopressors on the hepato- and splanchnic perfusion.

Although splanchnic perfusion may still be critical in sepsis, the endothelial dysfunction which accompanies these disturbances in vasoreactivity and perfusion, may limit the role of vasopressor therapy to alter the disease process. In the near future, attention should focus on effective treatments of vasoplegia and prevention of derangements of splanchnic perfusion in surgery and trauma.

References

1. Caldini P, Permutt S, Waddell JA, Riley RL (1974) Effect of epinephrine on pressure, flow, and volume relationships in the systemic circulation of dogs. Circ Res 34:606-623
2. Biffl WL, Moore EE, Moore FA (1995) Gut-derived mediators of multiple organ failure: platelet-activating factor and interleukin-6. Br J Hosp Med 54:134-138
3. Fiddian-Green RG (1993) Associations between intramucosal acidosis in the gut and organ failure. Crit Care Med 21:S103-S107
4. Kirton O, Windsor J, Wedderburn R et al (1998) Failure of splanchnic resuscitation in the acutely injured trauma patient correlates with multiple organ system failure and length of stay in the ICU. Chest 113:1064-1169
5. Hartung T, Sauer A, Hermann C et al (1997) Overactivation of the immune system by translocated bacteria and bacterial products. Scand J Gastroenterol [Suppl]222:98-99
6. Rombeau JL, Takala J (1997) Summary of round table conference: gut dysfunction in critical illness. Intensive Care Med 23:476-479
7. Davies MG, Hagen P-O (1997) Systemic inflammatory response syndrome. Br J Surg 84: 920-935
8. Fink MP (1994) Effect of critical illness on microbial translocation and gastrointestinal mucosal permeability. Semin Respir Infect 9:256-260
9. Takala J (1996) Determinants of splanchnic blood flow. Br J Anaesth 77:50-58
10. Anonymous. Third European Consensus Conference in Intensive Care Medicine (1996) Tissue hypoxia. How to detect, how to correct, how to prevent? Am J Respir Crit Care Med 154:1573-1578
11. Fink MP (1994) Effect of critical illness on microbial translocation and gastrointestinal mucosa permeability. Semin Respir Infect 9:256-260
12. Aranow JS, Fink MP (1996) Determinants of intestinal barrier failure in critical illness. Br J Anaesth 77:71-81
13. Lemaire LCJM, van Lanschot JJB, Stoutenbeek CP et al (1997) Bacterial translocation in multiple organ failure: cause or epiphenomenon still unproven. Br J Surg 84:1340-1350
14. Gottlieb ME, Stratton HH, Newell JC, Shah DM (1984) Indocyanine green. Its use as an early indicator of hepatic dysfunction following injury in man. Arch Surg 119:264-268

15. McLuckie A (1996) The COLD system of hemodynamic monitoring. Intensive Care World 13:24-28
16. Parviainen I, Ruokonen E, Takala J (1998) Dobutamine-induced dissociation between changes in splanchnic blood flow and gastric intramucosal pH after cardiac surgery. Br J Anaesth 74:277-282
17. Elizade JI, Hernandez C, Llach J et al (1998) Gastric intramucosal acidosis in mechanically ventilated patients: role of mucosal blood flow. Crit Care Med 26:827-832
18. Maynard ND, Bihari DJ, Dalton RN et al (1997) Liver function and splanchnic ischemia in critically ill patients. Chest 111:180-187
19. Jacobson ED, Linford RH, Grossman MI (1966) Gastric secretion in relation to mucosal blood flow studied by a clearance technique. J Clin Invest 45:1-13
20. Dalton JM, Gore DC, Makhoul RG et al (1995) Decreased splanchnic perfusion measured by duplex ultrasound in humans undergoing small volume hemorrhage. Crit Care Med 23: 491-497
21. Iince C, van der Sluijs JP, Sinaasappel M et al (1994) Intestinal ischemia during hypoxia and experimental sepsis as observed by NADH videofluorimetry and quenching of Pd-porphine phosphorescence. Adv Exp Med Biol 361:105-110
22. Pastores SM, Katz DP, Kvetan V (1996) Splanchnic ischemia and gut mucosal injury in sepsis and the multiple organ dysfunction syndrome. Am J Gastroenterol 91:1697-1710
23. Turnbull RG, Talbot JA, Hamilton SM (1995) Hemodynamic changes and gut barrier function in sequential hemorrhagic and endotoxic shock. J Trauma 38:705-713
24. Fink MP, Rothschild HR, Deniz YF et al (1989) Systemic and mesenteric O_2 metabolism in endotoxic pigs: Effects of ibuprofen and meclofenamate. J Appl Physiol 67:1950-1957
25. De Backer D, Zhang H, Manikis P, Vincent JL (1996) Regional effects of dobutamine in endotoxic shock. J Surg Res 65:93-100
26. Farquhar I, Martin CM, Lam C et al (1996) Decreased capillary density in vivo in bowel mucosa of rats with normotensive sepsis. J Surg Res 61:190-196
27. Lam C, Tyml K, Martin C, Sibbald WJ (1994) Microvascular perfusion is impaired in a rat model of normotensive sepsis. J Clin Invest 94:2077-2083
28. Garrison RN, Spain DA, Wilson MA et al (1998) Microvascular changes explain the "two-hit" theory of multiple organ failure. Ann Surg 227:851-860
29. Cameron EM, Wang SY, Fink MP, Sellke FW (1998) Mesenteric and skeletal muscle microvascular responsiveness in subacute sepsis. Shock 9:184-192
30. Wang X, Andersson R (1995) The role of endothelial cells in the systemic inflammatory response syndrome and multiple system organ failure. Eur J Surg 161:703-713
31. Curzen NP, Griffiths MJD, Evans TW (1994) Role of the endothelium in modulating the vascular response to sepsis. Clin Sci (Colch) 86:374
32. Avontuur JA, Bruining HA, Ince C (1996) Sepsis and nitric oxide. Adv Exp Med Biol 388: 551-567
33. Fink MP (1996) Does tissue acidosis in sepsis indicate tissue hypoperfusion? [editorial]. Intensive Care Med 22:1144-1146
34. Harris RA, Harris DL, Green DE (1968) Effect of Bordetella endotoxin upon mitochondrial respiration and energised processes. Arch Biochem Biophys 128:219-230
35. Schaefer CF, Lerner MR, Biber B (1991) Dose-related reduction of intestinal cytochrome aa$_3$ induced by endotoxin in rats. Circ Shock 33:17-25
36. Dahn MS, Lange MP, Wilson RF et al (1990) Hepatic blood flow and splanchnic oxygen consumption measurements in clinical sepsis. Surgery 107:295-301
37. Dahn MS, Lange P, Lobdell K et al (1987) Splanchnic and total body oxygen consumption differences in septic and injured patients. Surgery 101:69-80
38. Ruokonen E, Takala J, Kari A et al (1993) Regional blood flow and oxygen transport in septic shock. Crit Care Med 21:1296-1303
39. Friedman G, Berlot G, Kahn R, Vincent JL (1995) Combined measurements of blood lactate concentrations and gastric intramucosal pH in patients with severe sepsis. Crit Care Med 23:1184-1193

40. Olson D, Pohlman A, Hall JB (1996) Administration of low-dose dopamine to nonoliguric patients with sepsis syndrome does not raise intramucosal gastric pH nor improve creatinine clearance. Am J Respir Crit Care Med 154:1664-1670
41. Marik PE, Mohedin M (1994) The contrasting effects of dopamine and norepinephrine on systemic and splanchnic oxygen utilization in hyperdynamic sepsis. JAMA 272:1354-1357
42. Ruokonen E, Takala J, Kari A et al (1993) Regional blood flow and oxygen transport in septic shock. Crit Care Med 21:1296-1303
43. Levy B, Bollaert PE, Charpentier C et al (1997) Comparison of norepinephrine and dobutamine to epinephrine for hemodynamics, lactate metabolism, and gastric tonometric variables in septic shock: a prospective, randomized study. Intensive Care Med 23:282-287
44. Gutierrez G, Palizas F, Doglio G et al (1992) Gastric intramucosal pH as a therapeutic index of tissue oxygenation in critically ill. Lancet 339:195-199
45. Giraud GD, MacCannell KL (1984) Decreased nutrient blood flow during dopamine- and epinephrine-induced intestinal vasodilatation. J Pharmacol Exp Ther 230:214-220
46. Habler O, Kleen M, Hutter J et al (1997) Effects of hemodilution on splanchnic perfusion and hepatorenal function. II. Renal perfusion and hepatorenal function. Eur J Med Res 2:419-424
47. Bitterman H, Triolo J, Lefer AM (1987) Use of hypertonic saline in the treatment of hemorrhagic shock. Circ Shock 21:271-283
48. Oud L, Kruse JA (1996) Progressive gastric intramucosal acidosis follows resuscitation from hemorrhagic shock. Shock 6:61-65
49. Turnage RH, Kadesky KM, Rogers T et al (1995) Neutrophil regulation of splanchnic blood flow after hemorrhagic shock. Ann Surg 222:66-72
50. Johnson DJ, Johannigman JA, Branson RD et al (1991) The effect of low dose dopamine on gut hemodynamics during PEEP ventilation for acute lung injury. J Surg Res 50:344-349
51. Ward HB, Einzig S, Bianco RW et al (1982) Effects of dopamine and dobutamine on the myocardial and systemic circulation during and following cardiopulmonary bypass in dogs. Pediatr Cardiol 3:257-264
52. Chintala MS, Moore RJ, Lokhandwala MF, Jandyala BS (1993) Evaluation of the effects of dopexamine, a novel DA_1 receptor and β_2-adrenoreceptor agonist, on cardiac function and splanchnic circulation in a canine model of hemorrhagic shock. Arch Pharmacol 347:296-300
53. Donati A, Battisti D, Rechioni A et al (1998) Predictive value of interleukin-6 (IL-6), interleukin-8 (IL-8) and gastric intramucosal pH (pH-i) in major abdominal surgery. Intensive Care Med 24:335
54. Welte M, Pichler B, Groh J et al (1996) Perioperative mucosal pH and splanchnic endotoxin concentration in orthotopic liver transplantation [see comments]. Br J Anaesth 76:90-98
55. Bacher A, Mayer N, Rajek AM, Haider W (1998) Acute normovolemic haemodilution does not aggravate gastric mucosal acidosis during cardiac surgery. Intensive Care Med 24:313-321
56. Chang MC, Meredith JW (1997) Cardiac preload, splanchnic perfusion, and their relationship during resuscitation in trauma patients. J Trauma 42:577-582
57. Maynard ND, Bihari D, Beale R et al (1993) Assessment of splanchnic oxygenation by gastric tonometry in patients with acute circulatory failure. JAMA 270:1203-1210
58. Edouard AR, Dergremont A-C, Duranteau J et al (1994) Heterogeneous regional vascular responses to simulated transient hypovolemia in man. Intensive Care Med 20:414-420
59. Mythen MG, Webb AR (1995) Perioperative plasma volume expansion reduces the incidence of gut mucosal hypoperfusion during cardiac surgery. Arch Surg 130:423-429
60. Ruokonen E, Takala J, Kari A (1993) Regional blood flow and oxygen transport in patients with the low cardiac output syndrome after cardiac surgery. Crit Care Med 21:1304-1311
61. Kainuma M, Kimura N, Nonami T et al (1992) The effect of dobutamine on hepatic blood flow and oxygen supply-uptake ratio during enflurane nitric oxide anesthesia in humans undergoing liver resection. Anaesthesiology 77:432-438
62. Kaisers U, Pappert D, Langrehr JM et al (1996) Dopamine, dopexamine and dobutamine in liver transplant recipients: a comparison of their effects on hemodynamics, oxygen transport and hepatic venous oxygen saturation. Transpl Int 9:214-220

Metabolism and O_2 Consumption in Trauma and Sepsis

L. Brazzi, P. Pelosi, L. Gattinoni

Physiopathological background

Since its initial discovery by Priestley in 1774, oxygen was considered essential for life as it enables the energy contained in food to be converted into a form which can be used to maintain higher forms of life. The amount of oxygen consumed to continually oxidate the chemical substrate producing carbon dioxide is usually expressed as volume consumed per minute ($\dot{V}O_2$) and it is normally in the range of 100 to 120 mL $*$ min^{-1} $*$ m^{-2} or 200 mL $*$ min^{-1} for a typical 70 kg adult man. Oxygen is normally delivered from the lung to the systemic tissues by means of the blood and its amount is the product of the oxygen content of arterial blood (20 mL $*$ dL^{-1}) times the cardiac output (5 L $*$ min^{-1}), i.e. 20 mL $*$ dL^{-1} $*$ 5 L $*$ min^{-1} = 1000 mL $*$ min^{-1} (DO_2). The relationship between $\dot{V}O_2$ and DO_2 represents one of the most interesting autoregulating system in homeostasis since if one of the three components of DO_2, that is O_2 tension and haemoglobin concentration in arterial blood or systemic cardiac output, is abnormal, endogenous mechanisms are activated to regulate the other two in the way that normal DO_2 can be restored. Under normal circumstances, oxygen is present, within the mitochondria, at concentrations far in excess of that required to maintain its oxidative function and even if DO_2 decreases for any reason, $\dot{V}O_2$ remains stable over a wide range of DO_2 while the O_2 extraction, i.e. the ratio between the arterio-venous O_2 difference and the arterial O_2 content, increases (DO_2-$\dot{V}O_2$ independency). If the oxygen supply is reduced below a critical value, $\dot{V}O_2$ starts to fall as the O_2 extraction reaches its maximal level and the $\dot{V}O_2$ starts to be dependent on DO_2 (DO_2-$\dot{V}O_2$ dependency). In this situation, the local oxygen concentration could become inadequate to deal with the flux of reducing equivalent generated by intermediary metabolism and cell energetic processes can be limited by the lack of energy supply. As long as the limitation is restricted to facultative cellular function, the organ system function simply deteriorates; when also the cellular obligatory functions fail, cell homeostasis is threatened and irreversible changes start to arise in tissue and cellular function.

DO_2-$\dot{V}O_2$ relationship

A large number of clinical studies have focused their attention on the relationship between O_2 delivery and consumption in patients with different forms of cardiovascular disease [1]. In the great majority of these studies, for almost all the pathological conditions considered, a parallel change in O_2 delivery and consumption (DO_2-$\dot{V}O_2$ dependency) was observed at levels of O_2 delivery where O_2 consumption is normally independent from delivery. This observation prompted clinicians to support the hypothesis that critically ill patients are often characterized by inability to appropriately extract O_2. Hence, higher level of DO_2 could be useful to reduce mortality and morbidity in this group of patients [2, 3]. This is mainly true for septic patients, in which the inability to utilize oxygen and other substrates brought to the cells is well known [4-6], but is also true for trauma patients due to the fact that trauma seems to interfere with the processes of tissue oxygenation [7, 8]. Let us consider these two pathological conditions more in detail.

Sepsis

The "sepsis syndrome" has been defined by Bone et al. [9, 10] as a systemic response associated with infection. It has been reported that, during sepsis, tissue oxygen requirements increase by more than 50% above the normal values and that, despite the observed increase in cardiac output and DO_2, a shift from aerobic to anaerobic metabolism occurs with the development of lactic acidosis [11]. Starting from this observation, Tuchschmidt et al. [12], in 1992, evaluated the effects of increasing cardiac output and DO_2 in 51 patients with septic shock randomly allocated to either normal treatment (NT) or optimal treatment (OT). They found that the mortality rate was 72% in the NT group and 50% in the OT group ($p = 0.14$). They concluded that "... outcome in patients with septic shock appears to be related to the level of systemic oxygen delivery" and that "... titration of therapy to increase levels of cardiac index and therefore oxygen delivery may be associated with improved survival...".

The tendency to supranormal haemodynamic values, which often implies high dosage catecholamine infusion, is potentially dangerous, leading to arrhythmias, myocardial ischaemia and infarction. In 1994, we designed a prospective, multicentric, randomized trial to evaluate whether a haemodynamic treatment aiming at supranormal values could decrease mortality and morbidity in an unselected population of critically ill patients [13, 14]. Patients were randomized to three different strategies of care, defined according to the goal they have to reach over a predefined maximum period of five days: normal cardiac index (CI) values of $2.5 \leq CI \leq 3.5$ L * min^{-1} * m^{-2} , in Group I; supranormal values of CI (CI > 4.5 L * min^{-1} * m^{-2}), in Group II; and mixed venous O_2 saturation (SvO_2) $\geq 70\%$ or a difference between arterial O_2 saturation and $\dot{S}vO_2$

lower than 20%, in Group III. The recommended sequence of intervention to achieve therapeutic objectives was, as suggested by Shoemaker et al. [15], volume expansion and cardioactive drugs as considered appropriate or until adverse reactions occur.

Looking at the data obtained in the subgroup of patients classified by the attending physician as septic (116 pts.), we found that the higher the DO_2 at ICU admission, the lower the mortality at ICU discharge ($DO_2 < 400$ mL * min^{-1} * m^{-2} = 70% mortality; $400 \leq DO_2 < 600$ = 59% mortality; $DO_2 \geq 600$ = 39% mortality; $p = 0.0145$). As a matter of fact, this observation supported the hypothesis that increasing DO_2 could result in a better outcome, but the final results of the study differed from the expectation. Indeed, in this subgroup of patients, probably due to the fact that the mean DO_2 at ICU admission was already higher than normal values (556 ± 188, 599 ± 264 and 605 ± 290 mL * min^{-1} * m^{-2} for Group I, II and III respectively; $p = 0.6958$), we observed only a limited increase in DO_2 values, even in the supranormally treated group, during the 5 days study period (602 ± 127, 659 ± 203 and 628 ± 152 mL * min^{-1} * m^{-2} for Group I, II and III respectively; $p = 0.3462$) with no beneficial effect on mortality rate at discharge from ICU (50, 48 and 68%, for Group I, II and III respectively; $p = 0.1503$).

Trauma patients

Since the aim of circulation is to deliver an adequate volume of oxygen at an adequate partial pressure to replace the oxygen used at the terminal oxidase of the respiratory chain in the mitochondria, in severely traumatized patients a number of factor could interfere with tissue oxygenation.

It has been reported that normal values of heart rate, blood pressure and urine output may be inappropriate as a resuscitation goal in severely traumatized patients since a lower mortality and significantly fewer organ failures have been observed in a subgroup of patients with higher than normal values of cardiac output and oxygen delivery [16].

To date there are two studies that qualify as randomized controlled clinical trials and specifically investigate whether this approach, when applied to traumatized patients, is able to improve survival [17, 18]. Fleming et al. [17] evaluated the effect of increasing oxygen delivery in 67 trauma patients randomly allocated to either the control group ($n = 34$) or the protocol group ($n = 33$) and observed a mortality rate that was 24% in the protocol group and 44% in the control group ($p = 0.08$). Bishop et al. [18] evaluated the effect of increasing cardiac index, DO_2 and $\dot{V}O_2$ in 115 severe trauma patients randomly allocated either to the control of the protocol group and found that nine of the 50 (18%) protocol patients and 65 (37%) control patients died ($p = 0.03$).

Data from the same trial described above [13, 14] and referring to the sub-group of patients enrolled in the study as "trauma patients" (116 pts.) showed that:

1. DO_2 values at ICU admission were significantly lower than those found in septic patients (521 ± 175 vs. 589 ± 254 mL * min^{-1} * m^{-2}; $p = 0.019$);

2. even if a trend toward a lower mortality rate for patients with higher DO_2 value at entry could be assumed, no significant difference among the three considered subgroup actually exist ($DO_2 < 400$ mL * min^{-1} * m^{-2} = 40% mortality; $400 \leq DO_2 < 600$ = 31% mortality; $DO_2 \geq 600$ = 28% mortality; $p = 0.5686$);

3. therapies aimed at supranormal haemodynamic values lead to increased DO_2 values, during the 5 days study period (617 ± 132, 631 ± 143 and 607 ± 160 mL * min^{-1} * m^{-2} for Group I, II and III respectively; $p = 0.7770$) in comparison with basal data (550 ± 186, 471 ± 142 and 547 ± 189 mL * min^{-1} * m^{-2} for Group I, II and III respectively; $p = 0.0795$) with no beneficial effect on mortality (21, 34 and 38%, for Group I, II and III respectively; $p = 0.2763$).

Conclusions

As reported above, the use of supranormal haemodynamic values as a target for treatment has been proposed either for septic or for traumatized patients. Data reported here do not seem to support the hypothesis that maximizing DO_2 in these pathological groups of patients does affect mortality. Even if a definitive conclusion could not be drawn due to the limitation of the existing data, it is important to underline that recently at least two reports evaluated the efficacy of this approach for the treatment of unselected populations of critically ill patients [19, 20] and both concluded that further studies have to be conducted in the field of tissue hypoxia, especially with the aim of evaluating supranormal haemodynamic targets.

References

1. Gattinoni L, Brazzi L, Pelosi P (1995) Increasing oxygen delivery in sepsis. In: Sibbald WJ, Vincent JL (eds) Clinical trials for the treatment of sepsis. Springer, Berlin Heidelberg New York, pp 299-314
2. Shoemaker WC, Printen JK, Amato JJ et al (1967) Hemodynamic patterns after acute anesthetized and unanesthetized trauma. Arch Surg 95:492-500
3. Shoemaker WC, Appel PL, Waxman K et al (1982) Clinical trial of survivors' cardiorespiratory patterns as therapeutic goals in critically ill postoperative patients. Crit Care Med 10: 398-403
4. Dantzker D (1989) Oxygen delivery and utilization in sepsis. Crit Care Clin 5(1):81-98
5. Groenveld JAB, Kester ADM, Nauta JJP et al (1987) Relation of arterial blood lactate to oxygen delivery and hemodynamic variables in human shock states. Circ Shock 22:35-53
6. Vincent JL, Van der Linden P. (1990) Septic shock: particular type of acute circulatory failure. Crit Care Med 18:s70-74
7. Niiniskoski J, Halkola L (1978) Skeletal muscle PO_2: indicator of peripheral tissue perfusion in haemorrhagic shock. Adv Exp Med Biol 94:585-592
8. Kessler M, Hoper J, Krumme BA (1976) Monitoring of tissue perfusion and cellular function. Anesthesiology 45:184-197
9. Bone RC (1991) Sepsis, the sepsis syndrome, multiple-organ failure: a plea for comparable definitions. Ann Intern Med 114:332-333
10. Bone RC, Fisher CJ, Clemmer TP et al (1989) Sepsis syndrome: a valid clinical entity. Crit Care Med 17:389-393
11. Rackow EC, Astiz ME, Weil MH (1988) Cellular oxygen metabolism during sepsis and shock. JAMA 259:1989-1993
12. Tuchschmidt J, Fried J, Astiz M et al (1992) Elevation of cardiac output and oxygen delivery improves outcome in septic shock. Chest 102:216-220
13. SvO_2 Collaborative Group (1994) The SvO_2 study. General design and results of the feasibility phase of multicenter, randomized trial of three hemodynamic approaches and two monitoring technique in the treatment of critically ill patients. Control Clin Trial 14:255-260
14. Gattinoni L, Brazzi L, Pelosi P et al (1995) A trial of goal-oriented hemodynamic therapy in critically ill patients. N Engl J Med 333:1025-1032
15. Shoemaker WC, Appel P. Bland R (1983) Use of physiologic monitoring to predict outcome and to assist in clinical decisions in critically ill postoperative patients. Am J Surg 146:43-50
16. Shoemaker WC, Appel Pl, Waxman K et al (1973) Physiologic patterns in surviving and non surviving shock patients. Arch Surg 106:630-636
17. Fleming A, Bishop M, Shoemaker W et al (1992) Prospective trial of supranormal values as goals of resuscitation in severe trauma. Arch Surg 127:1175-1179
18. Bishop MH, Shoemaker WC, Appel PL et al (1995) Prospective, randomized trial of survivors values of cardiac index, oxygen delivery and oxygen consumption as resuscitation endpoints in severe trauma. J Trauma 38:780-787
19. Richard C (1996) Tissue hypoxia. How to detect, how to correct, how to prevent? Intens Care Med 22:1250-1257
20. Heyland DK, Cook DJ, King D et al (1996) Maximizing oxygen delivery in critically ill patients: a methodologic appraisal of the evidence. Crit Care Med 24:517-524

Intragastric pH (ipH) and $PaCO_2$ Monitoring in Sepsis

D. De Backer, J. Creteur, E. Silva

For many years, haemodynamic management of patients with septic shock had consisted in restoring and maintaining global parameters of oxygenation such as oxygen delivery (DO_2), consumption ($\dot{V}O_2$), and extraction (O_2ER). However, some patients may still have splanchnic ischaemia [1] and global parameters do not provide reliable information on the adequacy of splanchnic oxygenation. Two factors could account for the development of splanchnic ischaemia. First, in the presence of reduced blood flow, the splanchnic region may be at higher risk of ischaemia than the other parts of the body. When cardiac output decreases, adaptative mechanisms favour the blood flow redistribution to the brain and heart, so that the splanchnic blood flow may be the first to decrease and the last to recover during resuscitation. Furthermore, the critical DO_2 is higher in the gut than for the whole body so that this area may be more sensitive to reductions in blood flow. Second, the gut mucosa is particularly sensitive to alterations in regional blood flow because of a decrease in PO_2 due to the countercurrent mechanism and a decrease in hematocrit due to plasma skimming. Gut ischaemia may have clinical implications as it has been implicated in the pathogenesis of multiple organ failure [2, 3]. Hence, it has been recently proposed that improvement of regional haemodynamics, or at least avoidance of splanchnic ischaemia, should be included in our resuscitation goals.

Measurements of PCO_2 in the gastric mucosa can be easily performed at the bedside and provides important information about the balance between oxygen supply and demand. Although tissue PCO_2 equals arterial PCO_2 during steady state conditions, tissue PCO_2 can increase in various conditions. The increased tissue CO_2 levels reflect either an impaired CO_2 clearance in low flow conditions (CO_2 being aerobically produced by glycolysis) or an increase in CO_2 production in tissue hypoxia (by intracellular buffering of excess hydrogen ions by bicarbonate). Various methods can be used to measure mucosal PCO_2, such as direct measurement by CO_2 electrodes or tonometry. Gastric tonometry is the most convenient monitoring tool and is more and more used in critically ill patients to measure gastric mucosal PCO_2 ($PgCO_2$) and calculate intragastric pH (ipH).

Measurements of ipH and $PgCO_2$ by tonometry

The technique was first described by Fiddian-Green et al. [4] and included a saline-filled gas-permeable balloon placed in the gastric lumen. After a defined time interval (30 min or longer), allowing equilibration of the saline solution with the gut intraluminal PCO_2, the sample is aspirated for $PgCO_2$ measurement using a conventional blood gas analyzer. Several problems have been associated with this procedure, including an important variability in the determination of saline PCO_2 depending on the type of blood gas analyzer used, the long time interval needed for gas to reach equilibrium in a saline milieu, and errors introduced by saline solution manipulations. As CO_2 measurements are more easy and reliable, gas tonometry had recently been developed. Furthermore, assuming rapid and free CO_2 diffusion between the gastric mucosa and the lumen, this methods allows a shorter equilibration time. In vitro and in vivo validation of this technique demonstrated that gas tonometry is as reliable and more rapid than saline tonometry [5].

Intramucosal pH (ipH) can be calculated by the Henderson-Hasselbach equation, using the $PgCO_2$ value and the arterial bicarbonate concentration (HCO_3).

$$ipH = 6.1 + \log (HCO_3 / PgCO_2 \times 0.03)$$

However, tissue and arterial bicarbonate are assumed to be equal in this calculation, but this assumption is no more valid when perfusion is reduced. Furthermore, ipH can reflect systemic acidosis only in conditions in which mucosal perfusion is adequate (i.e. diabetic acetocetosis, chronic renal failure). Also, $PgCO_2$ can be influenced by changes in $PaCO_2$. Hence, the PCO_2gap, calculated as the difference between $PgCO_2$ and $PaCO_2$, more specifically reflects the adequacy of gastric mucosal perfusion.

Alterations of ipH and PCO_2gap in sepsis

In experimental studies on septic shock, mesenteric blood flow has been reported to be reduced, unchanged, or increased, according to the model and in particular the type of fluid administration. However, mucosal blood flow is usually decreased [6-8], with a decrease in capillary density [9]. Various studies have reported that ipH progressively decreased and PCO_2gap progressively increased after endotoxin administration [10, 11] or peritonitis [12, 13]. The decrease in ipH was accompanied by an increase in mucosal permeability [7] and the severity of the histologic lesions was proportional to ipH alterations [6].

Numerous studies reported that ipH or $PgCO_2$ could be altered in septic patients. In septic patients these parameters are good predictors of morbidity and mortality [14, 15]. Maynard et al. [14] reported that ipH was more sensitive than global haemodynamic parameters. Recently, Friedman et al. [15] extended these results and reported that combined measurements of arterial lactate levels and iPH were better predictors of outcome than each parameter alone. Furthermore, data obtained 24 hours after admission were more discriminant than data obtained directly after admission in the ICU.

Although various interventions have been used to improve iPH or PgCO$_2$ in septic patients, none of these studies were designed to assess the effects of these interventions on outcome. In a prospective randomized study, Gutierrez et al. [16] reported that survival could be improved by iPH guided therapy in the group of critically patients in which iPH was within normal values on admission. However, the mortality was not improved during iPH guided therapy in the patients presenting a low iPH on admission. In another prospective randomized study, patients with trauma who increased iPH above 7.30 within the first 24 hours of admission had a significantly lower mortality rate [17]. Although further studies are required, these data suggest that preventing the decrease in iPH could probably improve outcome in critically ill patients. Furthermore, it seems logical to avoid therapeutic interventions that could decrease iPH.

Effects of fluid administration

Although fluid administration is almost unavoidable in the therapy of septic shock, the effects of fluids on iPH are not well studied. In experimental conditions, the administration of fluid failed to restore iPH [10, 11]. In septic patients, the results were more divergent. Meirer-Hellmann et al. [18] observed that fluid loading increased iPH in patients with sepsis but these results were not confirmed by other investigators [19]. In the latter study, iPH or PgCO$_2$ were not significantly affected by fluid administration, however PCO$_2$gap decreased in some patients. Furthermore, the response in iPH could not be predicted from changes in cardiac output. Hence, iPH should be measured, and the effects of fluid should be tested in each patient.

Effects of blood transfusions

Using red blood cells transfusions to correct anaemia, Silverman et al. [20] failed to increase iPH in septic patients. Moreover, Marik and Sibbald [21] observed contrasting effects on iPH, depending on the age of the erythrocytes. Mucosal pH increased only when erythrocytes younger than 10 days were transfused, whereas iPH decreased with older erythrocytes. These effects were probably due to decreases in erythrocyte deformability that occurred during prolonged storage.

Various synthetic haemoglobin solutions have been developed recently. In a preliminary report, Reah et al. [22] observed that a disapirin cross-linked haemoglobin solution did not affect iPH in patients with septic shock.

Effects of adrenergic agents

In physiologic conditions, mesenteric blood flow is increased by β-adrenergic and dopaminergic stimulation and decreased by α-stimulation [23]. The various adrenergic agents usually combine α, β and sometimes dopaminergic effects, so that their effects on ipH would differ (Table 1).

Table 1. Effects of adrenergic agents on intramucosal pH (ipH)

Dobutamine	Unchanged [20, 26, 33, 39] or increased [20, 35-37]
Dopexamine	Unchanged [1, 33, 34] or increased [27, 32]
Dopamine	Unchanged [26-29] or decreased [30]
Epinephrine	Decreased [36, 41]
Norepinephrine	Increased [30]

The response in ipH to adrenergic agents would also be influenced by the simultaneous use of other vasoactive agents, the volume status, the level of positive end expiratory pressure, and the underlying condition.

Dopamine

Dopamine affects all adrenergic receptors types. At low doses (< 3 mcg/kg. min), the predominant stimulation of dopaminergic receptors may selectively increase splanchnic blood flow, but as the dose is increased, these effects are rapidly masked by α receptor induced vasoconstriction.

In endotoxic shock, Schmidt et al. [24] observed that low doses of dopamine delayed the onset of villus ischaemia, and Germann et al. [25] reported that higher doses of dopamine increased gut mucosal PO_2. These promising effects were not confirmed in clinical studies. Dopamine, even at low doses, failed to increase [26-29] or even decreased [30] ipH in septic patients. Furthermore, gastric mucosal blood flow, assessed by laser Doppler, decreased [26].

Dopexamine

Dopexamine stimulates the dopaminergic and β-adrenergic receptors but does not stimulate the α-adrenergic receptors.

In various experimental model of sepsis, dopexamine increased mucosal PO_2 [25, 31] but the effects on ipH were not assessed. In septic patients the effects of dopexamine are more controversial. In some studies [27, 32], ipH increased during dopexamine administration, although it was not affected in others [1, 33,

34]. Interestingly, Temmesfeld-Wollbrück et al. [1] reported that dopexamine significantly increased mucosal oxygen saturation while ipH was not altered.

Dobutamine

Dobutamine acts predominantly on β-adrenergic receptors but also possess limited α-adrenergic effects.

In endotoxic conditions, dobutamine either prevented the decrease in ipH [11] or increased ipH [7, 8]. This effect was due to an increase in gastric mucosal blood flow [8]. In septic patients, Gutierrez et al. [35] observed that ipH increased in septic patients who had an initial ipH below 7.33. Similarly, Silverman and Tuma [20] indicated that dobutamine increased ipH only in the subgroup of patients with a low ipH. Other investigators also reported that dobutamine increased ipH [36, 37] or decreased PgCO$_2$ [26, 38]. This effect was still observed even if patients were concomitantly treated with other catecholamines [38]. Nevière et al. [26] ascribed this decrease in PgCO$_2$ to an increase in gastric mucosal blood flow. However, these findings were not universal as some investigators failed to demonstrate a beneficial effect of dobutamine on ipH [20, 26, 33, 39].

In summary, experimental and clinical studies indicate that dobutamine consistently increases mucosal blood flow and ipH.

Norepinephrine and epinephrine

Norepinephrine had predominant α- and limited β-adrenergic effects. Epinephrine combines potent α- and β-adrenergic effects, the β-effect being predominant at low doses while the α- predominates at higher doses.

There are very few reports on the effects of these agents on ipH, both in experimental and in clinical conditions.

In an observational study, Meier-Hellmann et al. [40] reported that ipH was not significantly different in patients treated with norepinephrine and in patients with severe sepsis who do not require vasopressor support. In prospective interventional studies including septic patients requiring vasopressors, Marik and Mohedin [30] observed that norepinephrine increased ipH while Meier-Hellmann et al. [41] and Levy et al. [36] observed that epinephrine decreased ipH. In summary, a still limited number of studies suggest that norepinephrine may improve and epinephrine may alter ipH.

Non-adrenergic agents

Prostacyclin may increase ipH in experimental conditions [42] and in patients with septic shock [39] but these results need to be confirmed.

The effects of nitric oxide (NO) on mucosal blood flow and integrity are complex. It has been proposed that NO could be involved in the development of mucosal acidosis [43]. However, NO supplementation had a protective effect on villi [44] and NO inhibition decreased ipH [45] in experimental conditions.

To our knowledge, there are no clinical data in sepsis. In critically ill patients, Braga et al. [46] observed that perioperative feeding with an arginine-enriched diet could increase intestinal microvascular blood flow and ipH. However, this diet was also enriched with other factors that could also influence mucosal blood flow.

Conclusions

The effects of these interventions on ipH are complex and may be affected by various factors. Hypovolaemia and anaemia should be avoided but fluid loading and red blood cell transfusions do not systematically increase ipH. β-adrenergic agents usually increase ipH whereas α-adrenergic agents have more variable effects. Dopaminergic agents may not be as beneficial as expected. Promising preliminary results have been observed with some other vasoactive agents.

References

1. Temmesfeld-Wollbrück B, Szalay A, Mayer K et al (1998) Abnormalities of gastric mucosal oxygenation in septic shock. Am J Respir Crit Care Med 157:1586-1592
2. Landow L, Andersen LW (1994) Splanchnic ischaemia and its role in multiple organ failure. Acta Anaesthesiol Scand 38:626-639
3. Mythen MG, Webb AR (1994) The role of gut mucosal hypoperfusion in the pathogenesis of post-operative organ dysfunction. Intensive Care Med 20:203-209
4. Fiddian-Green R, Pittenger G, Whitehouse WM (1982) Back-diffusion of CO_2 and its influence on the intramural pH in gastric intestines of rats. J Surg Res 33:39-48
5. Creteur J, De Backer D, Vincent JL (1997) Gas tonometry: in vitro and in vivo validation studies. Anesthesiology 87:504-510
6. Wollert S, Antonsson J, Gerdin B et al (1995) Intestinal mucosal injury during porcine faecal peritonitis. Eur J Surg 161:741-750
7. Fink MP, Kaups KL, Wang H, Rothschild HR (1991) Maintenance of superior mesenteric arterial perfusion prevents increased intestinal mucosal permeability in endotoxic pigs. Surgery 110:154-161
8. Nevière R, Chagnon JL, Vallet B et al (1997) Dobutamine improves gastrointestinal mucosal blood flow in a porcine model of endotoxic shock. Crit Care Med 25:1371-1377
9. Drazenovic R, Samsel RW, Wylam ME et al (1992) Regulation of perfused capillary density in canine intestinal mucosa during endotoxemia. J Appl Physiol 72:259-265
10. Vallet B, Lund N, Curtis SE et al (1994) Gut and muscle tissue PO_2 in endotoxemic dogs during shock and resuscitation. J Appl Physiol 76:793-800
11. De Backer D, Zhang H, Manikis P, Vincent JL (1996) Regional effects of dobutamine in endotoxic shock. J Surg Res 65:93-100
12. Desai VS, Weil MH, Tang W et al (1993) Gastric intramural PCO_2 during peritonitis and shock. Chest 104:1254-1258

13. Ljungdahl M, Rasmussen I, Raab Y et al (1997) Small intestinal mucosal pH and lactate production during experimental ischemia-reperfusion and fecal peritonitis in pigs. Shock 7: 131-138

14. Maynard N, Bihari D, Beale R et al (1993) Assessment of splanchnic oxygenation by gastric tonometry in patients with acute circulatory failure. JAMA 270:1203-1210

15. Friedman G, Berlot G, Kahn RJ, Vincent JL (1995) Combined measurements of blood lactate concentrations and gastric intramucosal pH in patients with severe sepsis. Crit Care Med 23:1184-1193

16. Gutierrez G, Palizas F, Doglio G et al (1992) Gastric intramucosal pH as a therapeutic index of tissue oxygenation in critically ill patients. Lancet 339:195-199

17. Ivatury RR, Simon RJ, Islam S et al (1996) A prospective randomized study of end points of resuscitation after major trauma: global oxygen transport oxygen indices versus organ-specific gastric mucosal pH. J Am Coll Surg 183:145-154

18. Meier-Hellmann A, Hannemann L, Schaffartzik W et al (1994) The relevance of measuring O$_2$ supply and O$_2$ consumption for assessment of regional tissue oxygenation. In: P Vaupel (ed) Oxygen transport to the tissues XV. Plenum Press, New York, pp 741-746

19. Silva E, De Backer D, Creteur J, Vincent JL (1998) Effect of fluid challenge on arterial-gastric CO$_2$ gradient in septic patients. Crit Care Med 26:A38 (abstract)

20. Silverman H, Tuma P (1992) Gastric tonometry in patients with sepsis: Effects of dobutamine infusions and packed red blood cell transfusions. Chest 102:184-188

21. Marik PE, Sibbald WJ (1993) Effect of stored-blood transfusion on oxygen delivery in patients with sepsis. JAMA 269:3024-3029

22. Reah G, Bodenham AR, Mallick A et al (1997) Initial evaluation of diaspirin cross-linked hemoglobin (DCLHbTM) as a vasopressor in critically ill patients. Crit Care Med 25:1480-1488

23. Kvietys PR, Granger DN (1982) Vasoactive agents and splanchnic oxygen uptake. Am J Physiol 243:G1-G9

24. Schmidt H, Secchi A, Wellmann R et al (1996) Effect of low-dose dopamine on intestinal villus microcirculation during normotensive endotoxemia in rats. Br J Anaesth 76:707-712

25. Germann R, Haisjackl M, Schwarz B et al (1997) Inotropic treatment and intestinal mucosal tissue oxygenation in a model of porcine endotoxemia. Crit Care Med 25:1191-1197

26. Nevière R, Mathieu D, Chagnon JL et al (1996) The contrasting effects of dobutamine and dopamine on gastric mucosal perfusion in septic patients. Am J Respir Crit Care Med 154: 1684-1688

27. Maynard ND, Bihari DJ, Dalton RN et al (1995) Increasing splanchnic blood flow in the critically ill. Chest 108:1648-1654

28. Meier-Hellmann A, Bredle DL, Specht M et al (1997) The effects of low-dose dopamine on splanchnic blood flow and oxygen uptake in patients with septic shock. Intensive Care Med 23:31-37

29. Olson D, Pohlman A, Hall JB (1996) Administration of low-dose dopamine to nonoliguric patients with sepsis syndrome does not raise intramucosal gastric pH nor improve creatinine clearance. Am J Respir Crit Care Med 154:1664-1670

30. Marik PE, Mohedin M (1994) The contrasting effects of dopamine and norepinephrine on systemic and splanchnic oxygen utilization in hyperdynamic sepsis. JAMA 272:1354-1357

31. Schmidt H, Secchi A, Wellmann R et al (1996) Dopexamine maintains intestinal villus blood flow during endotoxemia in rats. Crit Care Med 24:1233-1237

32. Smithies M, Yee TH, Jackson L et al (1994) Protecting the gut and the liver in the critically ill: effects of dopexamine. Crit Care Med 22:789-795

33. Reinelt H, Radermacher P, Fischer G et al (1997) Dobutamine and dopexamine and the splanchnic metabolic response in septic shock. Clin Intens Care 8:38-41

34. Trinder TJ, Lavery GG, Fee JPH, Lowry KG (1995) Correction of splanchnic oxygen deficit in the intensive care unit: dopexamine and colloid versus placebo. Anaesth Intensive Care 23:178-182

35. Gutierrez G, Clark C, Brown SD et al (1994) Effects of dobutamine on oxygen consumption and gastric mucosal pH in septic patients. Am J Respir Crit Care Med 150:324-329

36. Levy B, Bollaert PE, Charpentier C et al (1997) Comparison of norepinephrine and dobutamine to epinephrine for hemodynamics, lactate metabolism, and gastric tonometric variables in septic shock: a prospective, randomized study. Intensive Care Med 23:282-287
37. Esen F, Telci L, Cakar N et al (1996) Evaluation of gastric intramucosal pH measurements with tissue oxygenation indices in patients with severe sepsis. Clin Intens Care 7:180-189
38. Levy B, Bollaert PE, Lucchelli JP et al (1997) Dobutamine improves the adequacy of gastric mucosal perfusion in epinephrine-treated septic shock. Crit Care Med 25:1649-1654
39. Radermacher P, Buhl R, Santak B et al (1995) The effects of prostacyclin on gastric intramucosal pH in patients with septic shock. Intensive Care Med 21:414-421
40. Meier-Hellmann A, Specht M, Hannemann L et al (1996) Splanchnic blood flow is greater in septic shock treated with norepinephrine than in severe sepsis. Intensive Care Med 22: 1354-1359
41. Meier-Hellmann A, Reinhart K, Bredle DL et al (1997) Epinephrine impairs splanchnic perfusion in septic shock. Crit Care Med 25:399-404
42. Starlinger M, Jakesz R, Matthews JB et al (1981) The relative importance of HCO_{3-} and blood flow in the protection of rat gastric mucosa during shock. Gastroenterology 81:732-735
43. Salzman AL, Menconi MJ, Unno N et al (1995) Nitric oxide dilates tight junctions and depletes ATP in cultured Caco-2BB intestinal epithelial monolayers. Am J Physiol 268: G361-G373
44. Boughton-Smith NK, Hucheson IR, Deaking AM et al (1990) Protective effect of S-nitroso-N-acetyl-penicillamine in endotoxin-induced acute intestinal damage in the rat. Eur J Pharmacol 191:485-488
45. Offner PJ, Robertson FM, Pruitt BA (1995) Effects of nitric oxide synthase inhibition on regional blood flow in a porcine model of endotoxic shock. J Trauma 39:338-343
46. Braga M, Gianotti L, Cestari A et al (1996) Gut function and immune and inflammatory responses in patients perioperatively fed with supplemented enteral formulas. Arch Surg 131: 1257-1265

INDEX

acute respiratory distress syndrome (ARDS) 150

anaemia 189, 192

anaesthesia
 spinal - 43

analgesia
 epidural - 43
 postoperative - 43

anaphylatoxin 55

angiopoieton 79

anti-adhesion molecules 79

anti-TNF antibodies 25

apoptosis 76, 107, 117, 118, 155

bacteraemia 65

bacterial translocation 169

body temperature 147

bronchoalveolar lavage 58

burns 153

calpain 113

caspases 108, 119

catecholamines 28

cell death 107

cellulitis 81

cholangitis 81

Clostridium difficile 110

community acquired pneumonia 148

complement activation products 55

corticosteroids 28

cortisol 43

cytokine 25, 76, 153

diabetes 109

dibenzyline 97

digitalis 102

diphosphoglycerate 98

diphtheria bacillus 100

DO_2-$\dot{V}O_2$ dependency 181

dobutamine 175, 191

dopamine 174, 190

dopexamine 190

duodenum 170

E-selectin 55
 - ligand-1 56

emphysema 81

endotoxaemia 138

endotoxin 137, 172

epidural analgesia 43

epinephrine 191

ethambutol 124

etomidate 43

fentanyl 43

fever 157

genes 49

genotypes 49

glucagon 43

glutamine 127

glutathione 78, 119

Gram negative infection 137

gut 169
 - ischaemia 187

haemoglobin
 synthetic - 189

haemorrhage 169

Henderson-Hasselbach equation 188

hepatitis 81

Hodgkin's disease 124

human genome 50

hydroxyl radical 118

hypertension 109

hypertonic saline/dextran 97

hypoperfusion
 regional - 169

hypotension 147

hypovolaemia 169, 175, 192

hypoxaemia 147

hypoxia
 tissue - 169

ibuprofen 79

indomethacin 43, 79

infection 49, 65, 123, 137, 147
 Gram-negative - 137
 wound - 81

inflammation 29, 76, 123, 148, 157

intercellular adhesion molecule-1 55

Interferon γ 78

interleukin-1 24, 52, 55, 78, 149

interleukin-1 receptor antagonist 27, 52, 126

interleukin-10 27, 78, 149

interleukin-6 25, 149, 154

interleukin-8 149

intestinal permeability 169

intragastric pH 187

intravenous immunoglobulin 161

ischemia 49, 76
   gut - 187
   splanchnic - 187

kallikreins 76

ketanserin 126

L-selectin 156

lactate levels 147

Limulus polyphemus 140

Limulus test 140

liver 170

low molecular weight dextran 97

lung parenchyma 55

macrophages 55

mediators 128

mental status 147

methylprednisolone 126

metoprolol 44

mitochondria 183

MODS 121

morbidity 67

morphine 43

mortality 67

multiple organ failure 117

naloxone 126

neutrophils 111

nitric oxide 118, 157, 192

norepinephrine 174, 191

oliguria 147

organ
   - dysfunction 147
   - failure 49

oxidants 55

oxidative stress 157

oxygen 181
   - consumption 187
   - delivery 187
   - extraction 187

P-selectin glycoprotein ligand-1 56

PAF antagonist 78

pancreas 170

pancreatitis 103, 150, 153

penicillin 102

Pentastarch 131

pentoxifylline 131

perfusion 169

pericarditis 81

peritonitis 81, 148, 188

peroxides 118

peroxynitrite 118

PGE_2 79

pneumonia 81
   community-acquired - 148

poliomyelitis 100

postoperative analgesia 43

prednisolone 43

procalcitonin 74, 149, 150

promethazine 126

prostacyclin 191

protease 55, 119
   - inhibitors 126

Pseudomonas aeruginosa 127

Ringer's lactate 97

Salk's vaccine 101

sepsis 49, 65, 121, 147, 147, 153, 172, 182
   - syndrome 65, 147
   severe - 65

septic shock 147, 187, 189

septicaemia 65

shock 175
   septic - 147, 187, 189

soluble tumor necrosis factor receptor 26, 126

spinal anaesthesia 43

splanchnic
   - ischaemia 187
   - perfusion 169, 170, 174
   - system 169

spleen 170

stomach 170

sufentanil 43

superoxide dismutase 119

surgery 177

syndrome
    acute respiratory distress - 150
    sepsis - 65, 147
    systemic inflammatory response - 23

synthetic haemoglobin 189

systemic inflammatory response syndrome
    23

tachycardia 147

tachypnea 147

thrombocytopenia 74

tissue
    - hypoxia 169
    - injury 55

trauma 153, 157, 177, 183

tuberculosis 102, 123

tumor necrosis factor 24, 51, 77, 108
    - alpha 55, 149, 153
    anti - antibodies 25
    soluble - receptor 26, 126

wound infection 81

ORGAN FAILURE ACADEMY

Sepsi e insufficienza d'organo sono condizioni che mettono in apprensione chi prende in cura il paziente critico. Qualunque sia la natura dell'evento scatenante, esso viene ad alterare uno stato biologico frutto di una armonica proporzione di elementi in equilibrio e contrastanti. La biochimica e la fisiologia, la fisiopatologia e la biotecnologia applicata offrono alla clinica solo spunti di interpretazione degli innumerevoli meccanismi che stanno alla base della sepsi e dell'insufficienza d'organo; tali eventi singolarmente o in associazione sono tra le cause maggiori di mortalità nei pazienti degenti in terapia intensiva.

È giunto il momento di lanciare una idea stimolante; creare un "consensus" permanente di studiosi ove ciascuno porti il contributo del proprio sapere e sia disponibile agli scambi interdisciplinari. L'Accademia per lo studio della sepsi e dell'insufficienza d'organo deve propagarsi in ogni direzione, avere carattere itinerante, proporre modelli di studio e di ricerca utili per la prevenzione e il trattamento di una patologia e di una sindrome che condizionano l'iter clinico del malato critico.

ORGAN FAILURE ACADEMY

La septicémie et l'insuffisance d'organes représentent des conditions pouvant à bon droit engendrer un état d'appréhension de la part du médecin qui doit prêter ses soins au patient critique.

Quelle que soit la nature du déclenchement de la maladie, il en découle bien évidemment une altération de l'état biologique qui est le résultat d'un rapport harmonieux entre des éléments qui peuvent être, à leur tour, soit en équilibre soit en contraste. La biochimie, la physiologie, la physiopathologie et la biotecnologie appliquée n'offrent à l'analyse clinique que des éléments préliminaires d'interprétation des nombreux mécanismes qui se trouvent à la base de la septicémie et de l'insuffisance d'organes: les différentes pathologies en jeu, prises individuellement ou associées les unes aux autres, constituent les principales causes de mortalité chez les patients critiques soumis à traitement intensif.

Le moment est venu de proposer une idée stimulante, à savoir la création d'un "consensus" permanent à ce sujet de la part de tous les experts en la matière: pour ce faire, il importe bien entendu que chacun soit disposé à fournir son propre apport en connaissances et qu'il soit à la fois ouvert à tout type d'échanges interdisciplinaires. Aussi faut-il que l'Académie pour l'étude de la septicémie et de l'insuffisance d'organes se développe dans toutes les directions, qu'elle ait un caractère itinérant et qu'elle soit en mesure de proposer des modèles d'étude et de recherche utiles pour la prévention et le traitement d'une pathologie et d'un syndrôme qui influencent en bonne mesure l'évolution clinique du patient critique.

ORGAN FAILURE ACADEMY

Für den kritische Patienten behandelnden Arzt sind Sepsis und Organschwäche besorgniserregende Zustände. Unabhängig von ihrem Auslöser stören sie das biologische Gleichgewicht, das sich aus dem harmonischen Zusammenspiel widersprüchlicher Elemente ergibt.

Biochemie und Physiologie sowie Pathophysiologie, angewandte Biotechnologie bieten dem Kliniker nur Interpretationsansätze für die unzähligen Vorgänge, die Sepsis- und Organschwächeerscheinungen zugrundeliegen; allein oder in Kombination zählen sie zu den häufigsten Sterblichkeitsursachen bei Intensivpatienten.

Nun ist höchste Zeit, eine stimulierende Vorstellung zu wagen: Die Schaffung eines ständigen Gremiums, in dessen Rahmen die verschiedenen Forscher ihren Kenntnisbeitrag leisten und sich am interdisziplinären Erfahrungsaustausch beteiligen können. Die Akademie zur Forschung von Sepsis- und Organschwächeerscheinungen ist als fächerübergreifender, wandernder Zusammenschluß mit dem Ziel zu gestalten, Studien- und Forschungskonzepte vorzuschlagen, die zur Vorbeugung und Behandlung von den klinischen Verlauf eines kritischen Patienten beeinflußenden Pathologien und Syndromen dienen können.

ORGAN FAILURE ACADEMY

Sepsis e insuficiencia de órgano son afecciones que crean cierta inquietud al curar el paciente crítico. Cualquiera que sea el género del factor desencadenador, éste termina por alterar un estado biológico fruto de una proporción armónica de elementos en equilibrio y contrastantes. La bioquímica y la fisiología, la fisiopatología y la biotecnología aplicada ofrecen a la clínica solamente unas indicaciones para la interpretación de los mecanismos innumerables que están a la base de la sepsis y de la insuficiencia de órgano; estos factores por separado o conjuntamente se hallan entre las causas principales de mortalidad entre los pacientes que reciben terapia intensiva. Ha llegado el momento de lanzar una idea inspiradora; de crear un "consensus" permanente de científicos donde cada uno lleve su propio saber y sea disponible a los intercambios interdisciplinarios. La Academia para el estudio de la sepsis y de la insuficiencia de órgano debe propagarse en todas las direcciones, tener carácter itinerante, proponer modelos de estudio y de investigación útiles para la prevención y el tratamiento de una patología y de una síndrome que afecten el curso clínico del enfermo crítico.

АКАДЕМИЯ ПО ИЗУЧЕНИЮ ВОПРОСОВ СЕПСИСА И НЕДОСТАТОЧНОСТИ ОРГАНОВ ЧЕЛОВЕЧЕСКОГО ТЕЛА

Наличие условий сепсиса и недостаточности у органов больного вызывает немалую заботу у врачей, занимающихся лечением тех пациентов, которые находятся в критической стадии заболевания. Возникновение заболевания, независимо от вида причиняющего фактора, изменяет биологическое состояние данного органа, определяемое гармоничным соотношением взаимокомпенсирующихся элементов. Биохимия и физиология, как и физиопатология, представляют клинике лишь исходные элементы для интерпретации совокупности механизмов, вызывающих возникновение сепсиса и недостаточности у органов человеческого тела. Эти механизмы, действующие отдельно или в сочетании друг с другом, являются одной из главных причин смертительности среди пациентов, находящихся под режимом интенсивной терапии.

Перед нами стоит, поэтому, важная задача, т.е. создание постоянного комитета ученых, каждый из которых должен будет делать свой вклад в дело изучения указанных вопросов и способствовать межотраслевому обмену информациями. Академия по изучению вопросов сепсиса и недостаточности органов человеческого тела должна будет иметь "передвижной" характер, т.е. распространяться во всех направлениях, и разрабатывать исследовательские проекты, необходимые для профилактики патологии и лечения заболевания, обусловливающих клинический подход к больному в критической стадии заболевания.

敗血症及び器官障害アカデミー

敗血症及び器官障害は、重病患者を治療している者にとって、特に気を配る必要がある。これらの全ての症状を引き起こす原因というのは、生物学の調和の釣り合い及び対照によって作られた均衡の崩れによるものである。生化学、生理学、生理病理学などは、臨床医学において、敗血症及び器官障害の基本的な多くの原因の解明の糸口を与える。またこれらの敗血症及び器官障害は、単一もしくは結合し、治療中患者の多くの死亡原因となっている。

この様な状況のなかで、今、ひとつの考えを提案する時が来ている。つまり、皆が共同研究の場所として、それに参与し、意見を交わす事の出来る、ひとつの"コンセンサス"としての、学べる場を作る事である。この敗血症及び器官障害のアカデミーは、多方面に普及し、また世界各地を回り、予防と病状の治療及びその症候群による重病患者の臨床討議に関与する研究調査を提案していくものである。

جامعة دراسات تريست – كلية الطب والجراحة

المعهد المتعدد التخصصات للتخدير والإنعاش والعلاج المسكن

المدير : الاستاذ . ج . موكافيرو

اكاديمية دراسات التقيح الدموي والفشل العضوي

بسبب التقيح الدموي والفشل العضوي فان الطبيب المعالج للمريض في الحالة الحرجة . فبغض النظر عن الاسباب المسببة لها ، تكون النتيجة في كل الاحوال هي اختلال التوازن البيولوجي الطبيعي الذي هو ثمرة تآلف نسبي بين عناصر متوافقة ومتعارضة فيما بينها . إن الكيمياء العضوية وعلم وظائف الاعضاء مع علم دراسة الوظائف اثناء الامراض تقدم للمتخصص فقط مجرد افكار عن مختلف العمليات التي تؤدي الى التقيح الدموي والفشل العضوي التي تسبب بدورها ، منفردة أو مرتبطة معا ، الى اعلى معظم حالات الوفاة في حالات العلاج المكثف للمرضى .

لقد آن الاوان لطرح فكرة جديدة ومثيرة : تتلخص في خلق طاقم عمل مشفاعم من الباحثين في مختلف التخصصات ، ليقدم كل منهم مساهمة في محيط مجال خبرته ليضهما تحت تصرف التخصصات الاخرى . اننا نتوخى نشر معلومات اكاديمية دراسات التقيح الدموي والفشل العضوي في كل اتجاه ، بحيث تكون منطقة في كافة الارجاء لتكون نموذج للبحث العلمي الذي يرمي الى الوقاية والعلاج من مرض وعوارض مؤثرة على المسار الاكلينيكي للحالات الحرجة .

脓毒症与器官机能不全学会

治疗病情危急病人时,脓毒症和器官机能不全颇使医生焦虑不安.引起这些病症的不同种类的因素都损害一个由平衡因素和相反因素按和谐比例形成的生物状态.对于脓毒症和器官机能不全的许多病因的形成过程,生物学,生理学,生理病理学只能提供一些提示.这些因素无论是单独出现还是并发出现都是接受特别护理的病人的主要死因之一.如今我们应该提出新的建议,创造持久性的学者之间合作的机会,使每个学者能发挥自己的才能,推动跨学科的交流.脓毒症与器官机能不全学会要向各地推荐有益的研究方法来防治及处理对病情危急病人的临床过程产生决定性影响的病理状态或综合症.